MENOPAUSE

RAEWYN MACKENZIE is a journalist and feature writer, and worked for the New Zealand *Herald* for eight years. She has also worked on a number of television documentaries. For five years she was Education Officer of the Auckland Family Planning Association in New Zealand, and pioneered courses for women experiencing the menopause, many of whom have contributed to this book.

HEALTHCARE FOR WOMEN SERIES

Coping with Stress
Georgia Witkin-Lanoil

Eating Well for a Healthy Pregnancy
Dr Barbara Pickard

Everything You Need to Know about the Pill
Wendy Cooper and Dr Tom Smith

How to Get Pregnant & How Not To
P. Bello, Dr C. Dolto and Dr A. Schiffmann

Lifting the Curse: How to relieve painful periods
Beryl Kingston

Menopause: A practical, self-help guide for women
Raewyn Mackenzie

Successful Breastfeeding
Joan Neilson

Taking Care of Your Skin
Dr Vernon Coleman

Thrush: How it's caused and what to do about it
Caroline Clayton

Women and Depression: A practical self-help guide
Deidre Sanders

Women and Tranquillisers
Celia Haddon

Women's Problems: An A to Z
Dr Vernon Coleman

You and Your Caesarean Birth
Trisha Duffett-Smith

You and Your Premature Baby
Barbara Glover and Christine Hodson

HEALTHCARE FOR WOMEN

MENOPAUSE

Raewyn Mackenzie

Illustrations by Philippa Blair

SHELDON PRESS
LONDON

First published in New Zealand in 1984 by
A. H. and A. W. Reed Ltd., Wellington 3, New Zealand

First published in Great Britain in 1985 by
Sheldon Press, SPCK, Marylebone Road, London NW1 4DU

Second impression 1987

Thanks are due to Pergamon Press Ltd., for permission to
reproduce the Holmes-Rahe Social Readjustment Rating
Scale from the Journal of Psychosomatic Research, Vol. II
(1967), pp. 213–218.

British Library Cataloguing in Publication Data

Mackenzie, Raewyn
    Menopause.—(Healthcare for women)
    1. Menopause
    I. Title   II. Series
    612'.665   RG186

    ISBN 0-85969-473-9
    ISBN 0-85969-474-7 Pbk

    Typeset by Photobooks (Bristol) Ltd
        Printed in Great Britain by
    Richard Clay Ltd, Bungay, Suffolk

Contents

	Acknowledgements	vii
1	Why a book on menopause?	1
2	How do you know when you're there?	8
3	The symptoms of menopause	19
4	The medical options	39
5	Contraception	46
6	Sexuality	52
7	Food for thought	69
8	Stress	82
9	Exercise	91
10	Cancer	96
11	How to set up your own menopause group	101
	References	109
	Index	113

Acknowledgements

My thanks to the following people for their help with this book: Shirley Child, Ngaire Irwin, Dr Tree Cocks, Heather Hutton, Leteia Potter, Janine Race, Christine Taylor, Dr Margaret Tillott, Barbara Kay, Gill Burrell, the volunteers and staff members of Family Planning, Auckland Branch, Betsy Marshall and John Gaiser, Cancer Society, Auckland Division, Cheryle Love and Virginia Shaw.

My special thanks to Maria E. Thomson for the many hours she spent on the diet section of this book and for her support while I was writing it; Dr Alison Riddell for her contribution to the contraceptive section, and Professor John Hutton for providing access to research material, for checking information and for his good humour.

But most of all, my thanks go to Claire Patterson, Deborah Harding, Edna Butterworth and Candis Craven, without whom this book would never have been finished.

Lastly, I want to thank all of the women from our sessions who contributed their experiences to this book. I know how difficult and sometimes painful it was to talk about some of the things we discussed. I hope that between us we have produced something which will make it easier for other women to talk about—and understand—this part of their lives.

ONE

Why a Book on Menopause?

This title should really be turned around. Why aren't there more books on menopause? All women go through menopause and women are hardly a newly discovered species.

The need for a book on menopause became apparent several years ago when I started running courses in New Zealand for women going through menopause and, along with other Family Planning Association staff, I went through the libraries and bookshops in search of good reference books. There were shelves of books on cooking, photography and just about everything else you could possibly want to know about. But on menopause there was little. What there was had a heavily medical bias, was outdated, distorted and often patronizing. The overwhelming feeling from the books available was that women who suffered from the symptoms of menopause usually had too much time on their hands and were basically suffering from not enough to do. In the end, we decided to order two books which women could buy from us. I'm pleased to see that these two are now stocked in a number of libraries—though I don't believe they would have been stocked had it not been for the demand created by the more than 2000 women who have gone through our courses.

So why is it hard to find the kind of information we want on our library and bookshop shelves? And where else do we go for the information that we need?

I think the answer to the first question is that menopause is not important to the mainstream of our society—mainstream meaning men. As to where to go for information—the first people that spring to mind are our doctors . . .

Rather unfairly, we've always regarded doctors as the source of all knowledge where our bodies are concerned. And, rather unfairly, they have accepted and reinforced that view. Again, doctors are often men and during their training they are given little information on the subject of

1

menopause. Menopause comes up informally in other areas, but coverage of the subject is inevitably haphazard. Moreover, doctors, because they are trained to treat *illness*, still see menopause as an illness. Perhaps unwittingly, we've colluded with that, and many of us expect 'cures' in the form of pills. If a doctor implies that the menopause changes which we are experiencing are all in our heads, then we will often accept that. Yet menopause is no more an 'illness' than puberty.

The logical people to whom to turn are our mothers, our sisters and friends who may already have gone through menopause. But even women regard menopause as a subject which, if it must be discussed at all, should be discussed in hushed tones. A striking example of this happened recently. One of our speakers on menopause had been invited to address the women members of a large club which also has a large number of men. The woman organizer explained to our speaker that, although the address was for women members only, it would be advertised on a noticeboard which would be seen by a large number of men. She was thus asked to describe the subject of her talk—menopause—as 'the problems of the mature years'.

Our fears about the reaction men will have to menopause —or to anything specifically to do with a woman's anatomy —are real enough. Two more examples of the sort of reactions we can expect come to mind.

The first happened some years ago when I was a trainee journalist. Within an hour of writing and handing in a story about cervical cancer, the editor had passed a surreptitious note to the subeditor who in turn directed that I 'note the contents'. The note said: 'The word cervix will never be used in this newspaper'. How we were supposed to write stories about cervical cancer without using the word cervix beats me!

Similarly, in 1981 I was involved with running a series of menopause courses which attracted the interest of various women reporters, one of whom was promptly called to the office of the editor and told that 'menopause is not a subject which people want to read about over breakfast'.

Secrecy and euphemisms abound whenever the subject of menopause is raised simply because we're still embar-

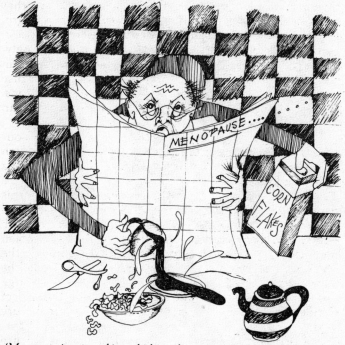

'Menopause is not a subject which people want to read about over breakfast'.

rassed, still ashamed and still feel fearful about bringing the topic out into the open. Much of our embarrassment can be traced back to the feelings we have about our bodies, and about menstruation in particular. As a teenager I used to walk the whole high street in search of a friendly looking shop assistant from whom I could buy sanitary towels. Most of my friends have had similar experiences. For all of us, menstruation, more than anything else, is a taboo subject.

Still, it's hardly surprising that menstruation should be seen as embarrassing, for punitive warnings about the mystical properties of menstrual blood have been hanging around for centuries. Its powers have been boundless—and often disastrous. Women could cause tobacco crops to become diseased in New Guinea; the fish to die in one of the Torres Straits islands; the rice crops to fail in Sumatra, and the cattle to die in some parts of Africa.[1]

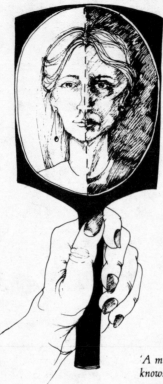

'A moment comes when a woman knows she has aged. This is the moment of menopause.'

In Maori lore, for example, women could neither prepare ovens nor cook certain kinds of food while menstruating. If they tried to gather shellfish while menstruating, they would all shift to another part of the coast. They were prevented from working in the sugar refineries of France because their presence would turn the sugar black! They were barred from Mexican silver mines because the ore would disappear. And should they have worked in the opium industry of Indochina, the sweet dreams of opium smokers might have become nightmares, for their presence would turn the opium bitter. More recent references give them the power of blunting razors, dimming mirrors and souring beer. Such are the powers of menstruating women!

But an equally big reason for not wanting to bring the subject of menopause out into the open is our anxiety about the implications of ageing—and menopause and ageing are inseparable:

> Women in this society don't want to get old for many reasons. We do not want to face the implications of ageing and therefore refuse to face the image of ourselves as having aged. But a moment comes when a woman knows she has aged. This is the moment of menopause.[2]

April showers, as the song goes, are for the very young. And so, according to the myths, are male adoration, lovers and anything else to do with sexual relationships. And if it's hard for young people to get jobs these days, that's always been the case for older women.

Our worth, as judged by our culture, is attached to youth, physical beauty and the bearing of children. We are judged against the 'perfect' women of the media—the Marilyn Monroes and Doris Days of past years; the Farrah Fawcetts and Bo Dereks of today. They're the young, beautiful women whom we see frolicking in the Club Med ads or being given roses by elegant young men in the Smirnoff pictures. We see only middle-aged women in the ads for oven cleaners.

To achieve the 'perfect woman' image is unfair to most women—and impossible for older women. But with the bombardment of 'perfect woman' images all around us, we can't escape the pressure to try and shape up to them. It's virtually inevitable that even we might start to believe that older women aren't worth much.

Again, this isn't just something which has arrived with the advent of high-technology media. Our history and our language are riddled with derogatory images of older women—the hags, crones and wart-covered witches of childhood stories are only a few examples of how deep this image of older women runs.

Now a new term has come to light in our language—ageism. It's a sign that women, seeing the discrimination they face because of their age, have started to react. In 1980 a new group was formed in the United States. Called OWL (the Older Women's League), the group was formed to fight discrimination against older women in US public policy. It has since become a vocal group on issues such as the re-entry of older women into the workforce and crime against older women. The group is saying, to anyone who'll listen, 'We matter'.

The first hesitant calls from older women started coming through to our department in the Family Planning Association in New Zealand in 1980. Family Planning is basically a contraceptive agency but it has also recently started an education division, in which I and some of the contributors to this book all work. Our receptionists, feeling that at last there was a department to which they could start steering the callers enquiring about menopause, did so, thinking that at least we might be able to refer women to useful books.

During the early months of 1980 the calls built up. Women who started by talking fairly superficially about menopause invariably got into deeper discussions, and gradually a picture of the less tangible signs of menopause began to become apparent: bouts of depression, bursts of energy matched by equally overwhelming bouts of lethargy, as well as the more commonly known hot flushes and sweats. Then in mid-1980 two of us were asked to take part in a radio talkback show about contraception. Somewhere during the programme a woman phoned in and asked about menopause—and then the floodgates opened. Every call from then on was about menopause. We realized that there were large numbers of women who desperately wanted information and had nowhere to go to find it.

We decided that we would start running sessions on the subject—short, three-hour sessions to which women could come to find out some of the facts they sought. As soon as the first session was advertised on the radio, our phones started ringing—non-stop. On some days our lines were so busy we'd get calls from the Post Office to say that people were asking that our phones be checked because they could simply not get through.

Our first session was a moving experience. We were all conscious of the fact that this session had a pioneering quality to it. Gradually the session took on a festive air, and when we broke for coffee we realized that the main worth of this—and subsequent sessions—was that women were talking to each other. The coffee break lasted for more than an hour. Some of the women in that first group formed friendships of long standing, and others have become involved with our later courses. Some of them still come to visit, and one of them helped with this book.

The sessions are still running—with greater numbers than ever and with just as many phone calls coming through whenever we do another advertising campaign. More than 2000 women have been through the courses, and around the country similar groups have been set up by our other branches and by various women's groups to whom we have supplied information on how to run the sessions. We have, too, done many talkback sessions since the one in 1980 and have provided speakers for many seminars. Menopause's time is coming.

This book has grown out of all those experiences. I sent out questionnaires to about 500 women asking them about their experiences of menopause—how long their symptoms lasted, which symptoms affected them most and how they thought that menopause had affected their lives, their sexuality and their relationships with other people. Over 300 women replied, and it is from their responses and from lengthier interviews with some of the women that much of the material for this book comes.

TWO

How Do You Know When You're There?

When we first started running the menopause sessions at Family Planning, we were faced with a dilemma. Would we make the sessions exclusively for women who were already going through menopause, or would we include women who thought that they were not yet in menopause but were wanting to arm themselves with facts ahead of time?

I decided that a proportion of mainly menopausal women to a few non-menopausal women was probably the right mix. The inclusion of too many women who had not yet been through menopause would mean that the women who were experiencing it would be in the spotlight, with the others placed in a passive or even voyeuristic role—listening but unable to contribute. However, as I had to have some way of screening who was or who wasn't going through menopause, I had to ask each woman who phoned to book for a session: 'Do you think you are in menopause?' If she said yes, I would then ask *why* she thought she was.

About half the callers said that yes, they were definitely starting menopause. They were usually in the 45-plus age group and were either beginning to experience erratic periods or had stopped menstruating altogether. Most of the remaining callers, however, did not know whether they were. Instead, they would ask *me* for help in identifying the early signs of menopause. How would they know what the signs were? It was a murky area. Some women said they had noticed increased discomfort before their periods; others said that they felt irritable. Some said they had started experiencing hot flushes, even though their periods were as regular as ever. Still others said they wouldn't be able to identify symptoms until they'd heard the experiences of others in the group and could compare those experiences with their own.

In the end, we decided that when in doubt, women should be able to come to the sessions unless they were very young and nowhere near the most likely age for menopause to

8

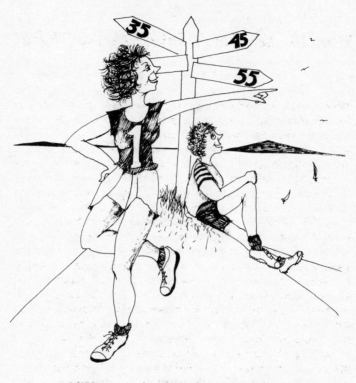

Menopause . . . how do you know when you're there?

begin—in the mid-40s to mid-50s. Even then we had to be very careful because some of the younger women seemed to show very definite signs of menopause. Sometimes, when questioned further, these women revealed that they had had total hysterectomies which had thrown them into an early menopause. The link between hysterectomy and menopause is discussed in Chapter 4.)

The medical profession defines menopause as 'the cessation of periods'—a definition which is semantically correct, since it accords with the original Greek meaning of the word, but which also seems to suggest that when your periods stop, that's that—that's menopause over and done with. Menopause is not that simple.

Some of the women in our groups have said that when they told their doctors that they had not stopped menstruating, the doctors had assumed that symptoms which had been bothering them were not attached to menopause. In fact, women themselves tend to define menopause not as the single event of their last period but as the entire transition time between the first vague signs of bodily change to the end of those noticeable symptoms. This 'transition' period can sometimes last from three to five years, or even longer in some cases.

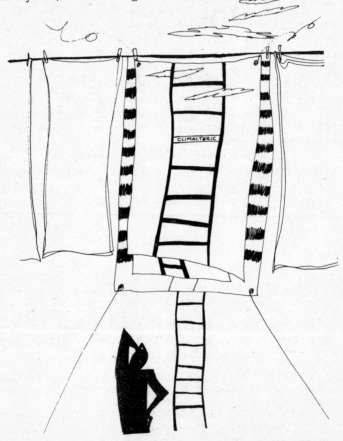

The word climacteric originally meant the step or rung of a ladder. This puts menopause into its proper place in the framework of our lives.

In this book, I will use the word 'menopause' to mean that entire time-span. It is a much more realistic use of the word.

The word 'climacteric' is another term still used quite often to describe this period of our lives. The origins of the word are Greek, and in its original context it meant 'step or rung of a ladder'—which to me puts menopause into its proper place in the framework of our lives.

The signs

The most common early sign of entry into menopause is the experience of erratic periods. They may be lighter, heavier, come earlier, or come at irregular intervals. Another common sign is unusual swings in mood. Sharp fluctuations in mood are a characteristic pattern in menopause, but these mood swings can also be complicated by the changes in lifestyle which often also occur at this time.

Hot flushes are of course another of the early signs, and may be experienced for anything up to two or three years before periods actually stop.

Any one or a combination of these symptoms can mean that you're into the onset of menopause. Here are some of the replies given when I asked women in our sessions what their first signs of menopause were:

The first signs for me were different patterns in my periods. I've always had regular periods, usually lasting seven days, but these began to be every three weeks or so and lasted only three days.

My periods became erratic; I started to get hot flushes; waking up in the night and not being able to breathe.

My monthly flow lessened and then my periods ceased. I had pre-menstrual tension until I could scream, and other days I couldn't have cared less about anything.

I felt moody and a general resentment at life. I felt that everyone was making it except me.

I started to get very agitated and tizzy—almost panic-stricken at times, even over minor things.

Lighter blood loss and bouts of aching bones, and deep misery at and just before my period and during the first two days of it. I

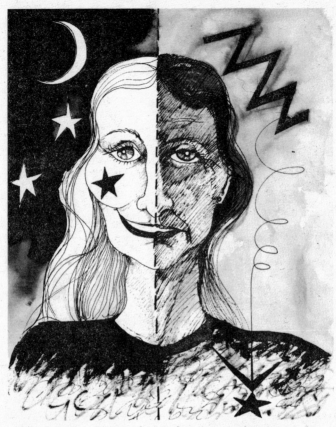

Sharp fluctuations in mood are a characteristic pattern in menopause.

was weeping over nothing when normally I'm a calm, cheerful person.

When I was 48 I didn't have a period for three months. I felt less anger and more relaxed than usual—but less energetic.

My periods became scantier, but lingered for seven to ten days. Then I would miss a cycle altogether for a month or two. I started getting night sweats, hot flushes and feelings of inadequacy and indecisiveness—feeling that I wasn't needed.

My periods were erratic and sometimes I had flooding. I got depressed and inward-thinking the day before my periods, and

I became extremely forgetful. I was most embarrassed to have totally forgotten at least three appointments until it was too late. I've never had total blanks quite the same before.

I had minor hot flushes at intervals—nothing much.

I had changes in my periods. They were heavier, lighter, less frequent, more frequent for two years or so. I had hot flushes, and I expect that more frequent headaches—from severe to migraine—were also a symptom which I hadn't realised.

I had dizzy spells.

I noticed that my vagina was dry. My pre-menstrual tension was also bad.

So, although we eventually share the common experience of our periods stopping, each of us will have a different singular experience of first signs of menopause.

For those without the signs

If you haven't experienced any of the signs I've talked about, you may be wondering if there is any way of anticipating when you might go through menopause.

There does seem to be a relationship between the age at which your mother or older sisters went through menopause and the age at which you might also. You can therefore make some rough predictions by asking your mother, your sisters or your mother's sisters when their periods stopped. If you smoke, however, you may find that you get there before the anticipated time, for smoking seems to hasten the whole ageing process.

If you just want some sort of rough guide to the likely onset of menopause, each country has an average age, but anywhere between 45 and 55 is common, and earlier or a little later than that is normal, too.

There is also a common belief that a connection exists between the age at which your periods started and the age at which they will stop. It was thought that if your first period began early in life, then menopause would be later rather than earlier. There does not, however, seem to be any scientific support for this theory.

What's happening to us?

It seems obvious that women would find the climacteric easier
to live through if they had accurate factual knowledge about it.
This information is hard to come by.[3]

There are three clear physical changes associated with
menopause. Our bodies decrease the production of our two
female hormones, oestrogen and progesterone; our ovaries
stop producing eggs, and our periods stop.

It's stating the obvious to say that each of us has a body
which has the ability to become pregnant. At birth, each of
us has a full supply of unripened eggs in our ovaries (unlike
men who manufacture sperm as they go). These eggs will
start ripening sometime soon after our first period, then
will continue to do so until a year or two before our
menopause. As we approach menopause, most of our
stocks of eggs will have run out—and that seems to be one
of the triggering points for menopause.

But first I want to go back to the beginning. The stage of
our lives at which we have the greatest number of
unripened eggs is when we are a five-month-old foetus. In
other words, our peak is reached before we are born, and
from then on the eggs start to disintegrate. As a five-month
foetus we have between six and seven million eggs, and by
the time we reach puberty these stocks will have dwindled
to one-third of a million—still ample, because in our
reproductive period we'll need only about 450!

But this egg-ripening business between puberty and
menopause doesn't happen of its own accord. It's governed
by a network of hormonal controls. They come in three
levels in our body. The top part of the mechanism is in our
brain and is called the hypothalamus. I've heard the
hypothalamus described as the emotional brain in our
system, or—another way of looking at it—as the conductor
of the endocrine system. That's the part of our hormonal
controls which responds to a shock and can shut down our
hormonal system or make it do something unexpected if we
suddenly come under stress. So if we do get a shock—say a
car accident or a death—or even experience a less major
upset such as an exam, our hypothalamus can signal our
next tier of hormonal controls to shut off temporarily. That

can make us miss a period, or maybe start bleeding at a strange time of the month.

The second tier of hormonal controls is a little pea-sized organ at the base of the brain and is called the pituitary gland. It's really just a gland which produces hormones—chemical messengers which go from one place to another in our body, signalling the other parts to perform some duty. The pituitary produces quite a lot of hormones. Among others, it produces the hormones which make us grow. If someone is exceptionally tall, for instance, it may be because he or she has an abnormal pituitary gland. It also controls our thyroid gland, so sometimes if something goes wrong with our pituitary our thyroid might also malfunction and we might either lose a lot of weight and become very trembly and pop-eyed or we might put on a lot of weight and get very sluggish.

The pituitary also controls the third layer of our hormonal system—our ovaries. The ovaries, as well as storing all the unripened eggs, produce two hormones, oestrogen and progesterone. These two hormones act on a number of parts of the body. One part is our breast tissue. You may find that at different times between your periods your breasts feel tender or prickly and they may even change in size throughout your menstrual cycle.

Other parts of the body which respond to these hormones are your vagina and the entrance or mouth of the womb (the cervix). Quite often, about the middle of our cycle, we feel quite wet around the vagina. That's because at mid-cycle there is a lot of oestrogen in our system. This makes the vagina and cervix produce more lubrication so that it is easy for sperm to enter through the small hole in the cervix and swim in search of an egg to fertilize. And of course nature is very intentional about all these body changes, because it's at about this time of our cycle that we are going to ovulate.

Oestrogen also affects the urethra—the small passage directly in front of the vagina which goes up to the bladder. The lining of this is very similar to the lining of the vagina, and oestrogen keeps both of them moist.

Between them, our pituitary and our ovaries are the glands which decide when we are going to start our periods. It's believed that once a girl gets to a certain body weight, the hormonal system is tripped. (And as an interesting aside, girls are now more likely to have their periods earlier than in the past—because they now reach that critical body weight earlier.) Then, from puberty until menopause, with a couple of years at each end of the changeover, our bodies usually settle into a reasonably consistent pattern of hormonal behaviour.

The cycles

It was not until late in the eighteenth century that medical researchers hit upon the fact that ovaries were probably linked in some way to menstruation, since their absence or destruction resulted in the stopping of periods. But various misconceptions—for instance, that ovulation and menstruation happened simultaneously—carried on until the beginning of the twentieth century, and it wasn't until 1915 that it was discovered that all the endocrine glands are involved at menopause.[4]

The lack of knowledge about how these systems worked resulted in some interesting case studies. One doctor of the late eighteenth century gave one of the best that I can find. His patient, he said, first menstruated at 20. Her first child was born when she was 47 and the last of her eight was born when she was 60. Her periods then stopped, he recorded, but they started again when she was 75 and continued until she was 98. This time, so the story goes, there was only a relatively small gap of six years before they restarted again—at the age of 104. Unfortunately, documentation of this fascinating case stopped in 1812, when presumably the patient was still menstruating regularly.[5] Presumably, too, the case study stopped because the patient had outlived the doctor documenting her!

But back to our ovaries and the way our menstrual cycles do work.

Let's start at day one of our periods—and incidentally, when we're talking about cycles, that's the point at which any medical description you may read will start. From day one to half-way through our cycle, our pituitary gland instructs our ovaries to produce a burst of oestrogen. The purpose of this is to ripen one of the eggs in one of our ovaries and to start building the lining of the womb to form a food 'nest' if that egg is going to be fertilized. Around the middle of the cycle, the egg bursts out of the surface of one ovary. Waving fingers at the end of the Fallopian tubes pick up the egg and it starts rolling along the tube en route to the womb. If you think of the egg travelling along the tube as the yolk, the piece which would be white is left behind on the surface of the ovary.

In the second half of our cycle, this 'egg white' produces another hormone, progesterone, which prepares the womb for implantation by building up a spongy lining of food for the egg if needed. Then, in the last few days of the cycle before our period, if the egg is not fertilized both oestrogen and progesterone production drops. As a result, the lining of the womb starts to break down and this becomes our period. And so, on the first day of our period, our cycle starts all over again.

Throughout all those years when we're having our periods, the hormonal messages keep running from one hormonal tier to the other in a hormone circle. The hypothalamus kicks the pituitary into action; the pituitary makes our ovaries produce oestrogen and progesterone, and when enough has been produced the hypothalamus is signalled to stop prodding our pituitary gland.

At menopause, this chain of command starts to falter, for our ovaries no longer produce enough hormones to trigger.

Oestrogen

This doesn't mean that we will have no oestrogen after menopause. Although we will no longer have enough to build up the walls of our uterus and thus produce our periods each month, our ovaries will still produce smaller amounts of oestrogen. Oestrogen will also be created in other parts of our body. Virtually all women continue to produce some oestrogen for the rest of their lives.

You may remember the ups and downs you might have gone through at puberty—irregular periods, some heavy, perhaps some others almost non-existent. The physical and emotional peaks and dips we experienced then were all signs of hormonal 'teething pains' as our body prodded a new system into action. This pattern is repeated at menopause but in reverse, for the hormonal winding-down may also be a jerky operation. Sometimes the various hormonal tiers work slightly out of synchronization, and sometimes one of the tiers will make an attempt to re-establish the hormonal functions with sporadic bursts of hormones.

Some women, and usually those whose hormonal systems have slowed gradually, find that they have few problems at menopause. But others of us experience sudden drops and then accompanying bursts of hormones, and our bodies may act in a confused and deprived way until the transition back to a non-fertile state is achieved. According to surveys, about 80 per cent of us will experience some symptoms, but these are relevant only if they affect our lives to any degree.

The mechanics of menopause are one thing. The implications of it on our lives are another thing entirely.

THREE

The Symptoms of Menopause

One of the things that amazed me during our numerous menopause sessions was the diversity of symptoms experienced by women. At first, some of them seemed too unrelated to be menopausal, but the strange ones kept coming up again and again and in the end a pattern began to emerge.

Some of these symptoms are fairly easily explainable; others are less straightforward. But before we look at each one in more detail, you might be wondering how likely it is that *you* will experience these symptoms. This is hard to gauge, for most of the women who come to our courses do so because they *are* concerned or puzzled about symptoms and are actively seeking help in working them out.

A national health survey which was carried out in the United States between 1960 and 1962 estimated that about 16 per cent of all women won't have symptoms at all.[6] (One of the women I work with told me: 'One day my periods just stopped—and that's all there was to it. Not a hot flush, nothing.' I've heard this story frequently from others.) Nevertheless, the same survey gives a figure of 10 per cent for those women experiencing 'severe' menopausal problems, and also indicates that about 75 per cent of all women will experience some symptoms. As we've already seen, these symptoms are very variable and affect each of us in different ways.

About two-thirds of the women who answered the questionnaire I sent to them after our sessions said that they had felt they needed help, but only half said they felt they needed *medical* help. And even then their reason for going to a doctor was more to seek information and reassurance than to seek actual medication. Frequently, women have said that when given medication they did not take the pills:

I needed help from my doctor and my husband. I needed

support and understanding, and specific knowledge would have helped. But really what I wanted was just to know that someone cared and wanted to help instead of treating me as though I was being a nuisance. The doctor just gave me anti-depressants and said, 'Well, at your age . . .'

I'm not really one for talking about personal things to friends. My partner—well, he tries to be helpful but doesn't really understand. The doctor doesn't have time—he says to me, 'Try these pills, they'll help you to sleep.' I would have liked to have known if my monthly period stopping was the start of menopause. I would have liked to know if my moods and depressed days were normal—or if I was going around the bend.

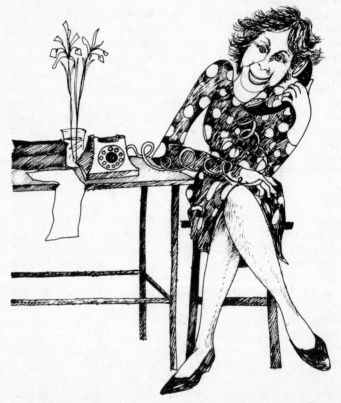

Over and over again women have said they needed someone to talk to.

> I needed medical help to make sure there was no disease and to have the onset of climacteric confirmed. I wanted to know what I could expect in the way of symptoms and changes to my body.

Over and over again the need for 'someone to talk to' was brought up:

> I felt anxious about the unknown. I felt I needed help, but only sometimes, and this was when I felt bad—sorry for myself. I couldn't pin down why I felt this way. My most supportive help has been from women friends my own age. We just compare symptoms and the telling and sharing seems to ease the isolation.

Physical symptoms

Physical symptoms are easier to talk about than emotional changes. This is probably why so many of the menopause books available spend much of their time talking about them rather than the emotions which surround them.

It's also the reason why I'm going to deal with physical symptoms first—even though they are not the symptoms which worry women most. In fact, mood changes, which include depression, anxiety, weepiness and feelings of panic, bewilderment and confusion were the symptoms most frequently cited when women were asked: 'Were there any aspects of menopause which you found to be a problem? Has it interfered with your day-to-day functioning ability?' After these mood changes came flushes; then came tiredness, then flooding, headaches, vaginal dryness (or vaginal discharges), wakefulness, memory loss, aching joints, flatulence and digestive problems, feelings of bloatedness, bladder irritation, vivid or upsetting dreams and loss of libido. Others mentioned less frequently were tingling sensations in the fingers and toes, and gum problems.

The three most commonly talked about—or at least the three most commonly known—symptoms of menopause are *hot flushes (and sweats)*, *vaginal dryness* and *osteoporosis*, which is a condition in which our bones start losing their strength and density. The first two of these are linked to the decrease of oestrogen experienced at menopause, and it is thought that osteoporosis may sometimes also be influenced by this. Flushes and vaginal dryness are the only two conditions which definitely respond to oestrogen treatment; it is effective in treating osteoporosis only in some cases. This is discussed in more depth in Chapter 4.

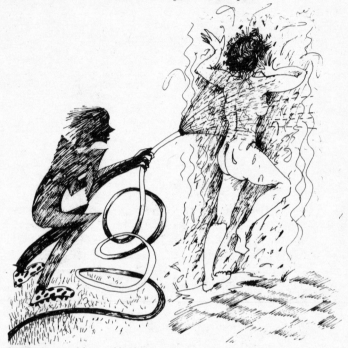

Hot flushes . . . like a sudden burst of water when you walk through the spray of a hose.

Hot flushes

Hot flushes—or hot flashes, as they're sometimes called— are variable. Women in our groups say that quite often they'll come in batches; sometimes they won't get them for months at a time. No particular pattern for predicting their appearance has been identified, however. Some women have said that they thought stress played a part in their appearance, but others have said that they got them 'at any old time' rather than at any particular time.

And everyone describes hot flushes differently. This is not the way they're usually described in books, which focus their occurrence in the upper breasts, neck and face.

I didn't know what it was like to sweat until I started having hot flushes. It was like someone turning a hot tap on me—like the sudden burst of water when you walk through the spray of a hose.

When I first started having hot flushes I would spend more time on top of the bed than under the blankets at night. In fact some nights I would think, 'I don't want to go to bed tonight, it's going to be one of those nights'. It can drench my nightgown. Once or twice I've got up and changed. But most of the time I've only been wet from the breasts up—it seems to be localized.

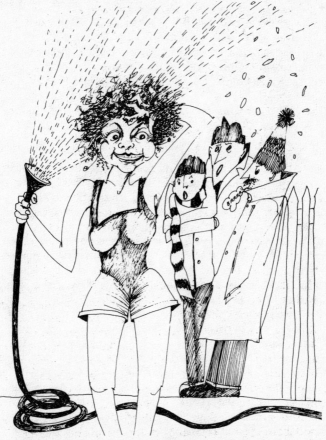

Some women said they welcomed hot flushes in cold weather.

These two cases are probably among the most extreme. Hot flushes can range from severe to quite mild, and some women have said that they had only the occasional hot flush and did not find them particularly upsetting. Others even said they'd welcomed them in cold weather!

In addition to the physical discomfort of hot flushes and sweats (and that includes the 'chilly sensations' which many women experience afterwards), they can be socially very embarrassing. In fact, many flushes *can't* be noticed by other people ('I've looked in the mirror, and that's true!'), but for many women the sudden onset of a hot flush in public can be disconcerting. It *feels* like everyone will notice.

Because the cause of hot flushes is still largely unknown, effective treatment cannot always be guaranteed. One woman said that deep breathing provided her with some relief; others have found that vitamin E or the use of cologne was helpful. We do know, however, that oestrogen treatment can have a dramatic effect in reducing hot flushing, and this treatment will·be discussed further in Chapter 4.

Vaginal dryness
When our oestrogen production drops, the walls of both our vagina and urethra thin down and become more delicate and fragile, with far less natural moisture than previously. This can mean painful intercourse. It's a relatively minor problem for many women, but it can be distressing if sexual intercourse is an important part of any relationship. It can also be a problem in that it makes us more prone to vaginal infections—and sometimes to infections of the bladder, since the urethra or the passage leading up to the bladder is not getting the higher doses of oestrogen each month.

Quite frequently women mention that they have 'an unpleasant odour' from vaginal discharges. This usually means that there is an infection which should be treated. Again, if you look in the section on oestrogen in Chapter 4 you'll see what is suggested. For vaginal dryness, KY Jelly, a slippery lubricant available from most chemists, can be helpful. For some women, regular sexual activity, whether with a partner or masturbation, has also helped to *keep* the vagina lubricated.

Osteoporosis

As we get older our bones start losing their density and strength. That's a natural process. The so-called 'little old lady' is called that because she has in fact shrunk: we can lose up to about 6.5 centimetres in height in the years after menopause. This diminishing bone strength is also the reason why so many women break bones easily in old age.

Normally we lose about 1 per cent of bone as a result of ageing (it can be the reason for aching joints), but sometimes after menopause we can lose bone at a rate of something like two per cent a year. Professor John Hutton, a Professor of Obstetrics and Gynaecology, estimates that 'about 25 per cent of women, perhaps, lose bone faster than they would normally do due to ageing'.

You can't regain bone which is already lost, but some medical sources think that oestrogen therapy might slow down the rate of bone loss. Professor Hutton cautions that probably only about a quarter of the women receiving oestrogen therapy will experience relief from osteoporosis.

Other symptoms

Flooding is one symptom which should always be taken seriously. If flooding to you means regular very heavy periods, which can't be controlled with sanitary pads, this could mean you probably have fibroids. If you get flooding for one period but not others, this may either be a result of your ovaries failing to produce hormones properly or, less commonly, of an early miscarriage. In either case, report the symptoms to your doctor.

In fact, all the symptoms which are outlined here could be caused by something other than menopause, so there's good sense in having them checked by your doctor just in case they result from something else altogether.

Headaches sometimes occur as a reaction to flushes and sweats. If you have the flushes treated, this might also alleviate the headaches. Some doctors prescribe a drug called Dixarit. This, too, can be helpful. Some women have said that taking vitamin B_6 has been beneficial. Take from 50 mg to 100 mg per day, always starting at the lower dosage first and working up to 100 mg if the lower dosages don't work.

Tiredness can be made worse by broken sleep and night-time hot flushes, and may be alleviated if those symptoms are treated. For some women the traditional hot milk drink before bed really does help them get a good night's sleep.

Memory loss also worries a lot of women, and although it is something that all of us face as we get older, particularly bad patches of memory and concentration loss can occur during menopause:

> One day I realised that I had put the dirty dishes in the cupboard. At work I'm starting to forget appointments quite frequently. It's very distressing.

This lack of concentration and loss of memory may be associated with changes to the blood vessels. When absorbed, some foods convert to chemicals which can affect the blood vessels. Cheese is one food which can do this, so avoid it if you can. Try to get regular exercise, which definitely has a beneficial effect, and keep lists of things you have to do ('. . . if I can remember where I put the lists', said one woman).

Loss of libido is complicated. So many factors influence the way we feel about sex that it's difficult to attribute a single cause to the loss of libido. It can be associated with depression, and it can also be associated with the wider loss of self-esteem which many of us experience as we get older. (More on this in Chapter 6.) But if loss of libido is clearly a response to painful intercourse, this may be the result of an infection which commonly occurs when dropping oestrogen levels decrease the amount of moisture in the vagina. Again, a lubricating jelly might be helpful.

Flatulence and digestive problems have been recorded as being associated with menopause for hundreds of years, but they can often be caused by things unrelated to menopause. So can vivid or upsetting dreams. Although these can be linked with depression, many of the women who experience remarkably powerful dreams say that they aren't conscious of feeling depressed at all. For some of these women, a regular daily intake of vitamin B_6 has helped.

A feeling of bloatedness is also quite commonly reported by women in our groups, and often happens in the week before their periods. The cause of this is unknown, but it may be associated with fluid retention in the abdominal wall, or with a gaseous distension of the gut.

Tingling sensations in the skin ('like ants crawling over my skin') is another symptom which some women talk about. Again, we don't know why this happens, but it does seem to go away if you are on low dosage, cyclical oestrogen. Similarly, aching joints, palpitations and feelings of panic are sometimes reported to us. The only help I can offer here is the reassurance that other women get these things, too.

The blues
As I've already said, depression, anxiety, weepiness, wakefulness and irritability are regarded by most women who come to our sessions as the major problems to affect their day-to-day functioning ability.

Some people discount the link between hormonal cycles and mood, but there are a number of signs which indicate that hormonal fluctuations do have an effect on our emotions. For example, when hormone production tails off just before our periods, many of us suffer from premenstrual tension. And it's also known that differing amounts of hormones in various birth-control pills can affect the moods of the user. (On the other hand, oestrogen therapy does *not* have any beneficial effect on these feelings.)

Some women say that these moods occur in a cyclic fashion, and that even after their periods have stopped they continue to happen at certain times of the month. One way of finding this out for yourself is to keep a diary recording how you feel day by day. You'll then be able to see whether your moods follow a recognizable pattern. It's also obvious that if you're having some of the other physical symptoms which are affected by changing hormone production—like hot flushes and sweats during the night—then you'll be suffering from broken sleep. This, too, can contribute to depression and tiredness.

But there are other, more complex reasons why many of us feel blue at this time. Menopause is literally a 'change of life', when old roles have to be re-examined and new ones embarked upon. That's a very stressful thing in itself.

I had a mixed bag of answers to the question: 'How did

you feel when you realized that menopause had started?', ranging from ecstasy to sadness to nervous anticipation:

I felt great, I've been waiting for this since I was eleven.

I felt elated and interested. I felt generally pleased that my childbearing days were over, and challenged that a new era was beginning.

I was pleased that I had no more worries about having babies plus the discomfort and inconvenience of periods.

Sometimes I would wake up in the morning and think, 'Oh God, another day.' I just wanted to pull the blankets back up over my head and never get out of bed.

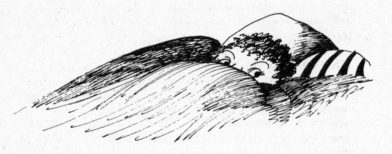

I had feelings of bewilderment, then of relief.

I felt my usefulness was over.

I was sad. I didn't want any more children, but it was so final—as if my usefulness had gone. It was quite a lost feeling.

I had very mixed feelings. My menopause coincided with my daughter's first period—she's 14, I'm 46. I was sort of lonely, had a lost feeling—this was a new stage of my life.

I had feelings of inadequacy—tiredness, forgetfulness. I felt emotionally unstable, indecisive, jealous, and I felt as though I was unattractive—just a ball of fat. One day I would feel fine, another day like this.

I was jubilant—the same feelings I experienced when the first signs of labour appeared.

Menopause and depression

We know exactly how society feels about ageing. In the last few years, along with terms like sexist and racist, we have come to recognize a new word—ageist, or being discriminated against on the basis of age.

Women are the victims of ageism. Look at the ads in magazines and on television. Thumb through a few magazines and look for the ads which represent middle-aged women. Try to find some positive images. They're simply not there—except in magazines such as the American feminist magazine *MS*. There are any number of advertisements showing glamorous women, but all of them are under 30. The pictures of middle-aged women show us in aprons and white smocks eulogizing about the benefits of washing powders. In her book *Women, Menopause and Middle Age*, Vidal S. Clay says:[7]

> The main thing a young woman learns in adolescence is 'to use the cosmetic exterior of the self to lure men, find affection and succeed in the competition of dating'. Girls are brought up to be weak, dependent and afraid of success (out of fear that they won't catch a husband). This is the way we are prepared for marriage. . . . Studies of women have shown that they have picked up the ideas about women that exist in our society. Even though people say they believe that our society is equalitarian, women, and men too, show more respect for the achievements and qualities of men. . . . Thus the majority of girls who were never taught or encouraged to be active, independent and assertive learn that they are important only when they are valued by men. A woman is not thought to be a complete human being by herself; she is believed to 'need a man' to round out her existence. Women are taught to get their main satisfactions in life from their relationships with men (and later their children) and they are expected to derive vicarious gratification from the achievements of their husbands (and children). Women are taught to live through other people. . . . How a woman responds to the notion of ageing and to the process itself depends to a large extent upon what she thinks of herself as a woman. If she feels she is valuable only when she is young and pretty then she is bound to have trouble with the climacteric and middle age.

There is no doubt that menopause represents a time for reassessing our attitudes to ourselves. Now is the time for us to think about *ourselves*—to put ourselves first—and since many of us have spent most of our lives putting *others* first, this switch is a big one.

Let's look at some of the things which are typically reported as happening about the time of menopause.

The end of menstruation
Our menstrual cycles have been with us for around 35 years by the time we reach menopause. And that represents a great deal of our lives. We may not have enjoyed having periods very much, but nevertheless they're an established routine, something that we've grown to live with. To some of us, the end of menstruation will represent a loss.

One of the women from our first menopause session talked about the way she reacted when she finally accepted that she was not going to have another period:

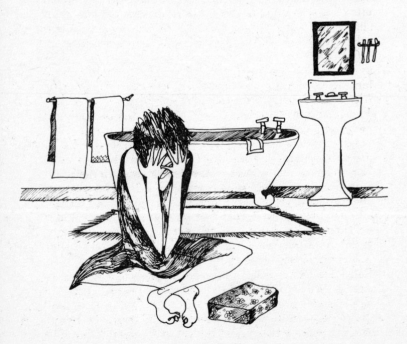

> I still had some sanitary pads left and had been meaning to throw them out for some time, since I no longer needed them. I went to throw them out and then I thought, 'No, I'll keep them—just in case'. I stood there with them in my hand, not knowing what to do. Then I sat down on the bathroom floor and sobbed my heart out.

And if the end of menstruation is one thing, what it means is another:

> It's a time of grief. It's a loss of youth. It's loss of the kids, even though it's time and sometimes I wish one was in America and the other in Siberia. We don't acknowledge this. All these things are happening. It's really hurting me—I need to have a damned good cry. We're not allowing ourselves time to grieve.

Loss of fertility

The end of menstruation means that we're no longer fertile. This is *not* the same as losing our ability to enjoy sexual relationships (though many of us fear this, given that we've seen reproduction as one of our major functions in life). Even if another child is the last thing we would want at this time, to have the choice removed is a major loss.

Loss of a job

Menopause often coincides with our children leaving home to lead their own, more independent lives. This creates what is pompously and patronizingly called the 'empty nest syndrome'.

There has been a lot written about the problems of retirement in magazines. But these articles are almost always about men and the stress that their changing of occupations can bring. Why is there so little around about how to cope with our 'retirement' from the role of mother? Quite simply, because child rearing is an unpaid job and is treated by our culture generally as not being a 'real job'. Therefore, if we're not doing a 'real job', we won't suffer from any stress when it finishes. Right?

Of course that's not right and of course we are going to suffer from all the things that other people changing occupations suffer. It's inevitable that many of us will experience genuine sadness when our children leave home. Over the years, raising our children has probably brought

31

us affection, cuddles and companionship. There are many real and satisfying aspects to raising children, even though the role has second-rate status in our culture. But many of us will also feel angry when the payoff for all the years of giving is 'desertion' by the very ones whom we've spent so many years working for. Again, a quote from Vidal Clay:

The accepted social role for married women today includes three areas—wife, mother and housewife. In middle age, some women lose the wife role, mothering is ended or will be shortly and only the housewife role is left. A major problem then facing

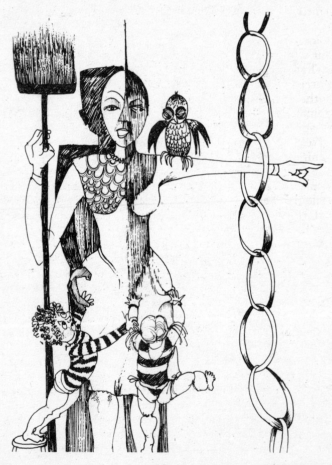

middle aged women who have lived the traditional home/
husband/child centred life is to find a new central role or
occupation themselves. Society has not prepared women for
this discontinuity in their lives.[8]

'When the children leave home . . .' How often have we
heard these words used as a justification for putting off
making decisions about our own lives? If we *have* been
putting off making these decisions about our lives, then the
time has now come for action. And that can be pretty scary
for us. Now is the time for us to re-establish our own
identity—without the props.

A new job?
'But what experience do you have, Mrs Jones?'
That phrase is enough to make most of us shrink with
apprehension. Don't we all know that our role of housewife,
mother, manager of household expenses, organizer extraordinaire and arbiter of disputes counts for nothing when
we apply for a job in the paid workforce?
We know that there's quite a chance of being discriminated against in employment—by people who think
that women should not compete with men and young
people for jobs, as well as by employers themselves. But
while it's difficult to beat attitudes, it's a mistake to think
that the many skills we've acquired over the years are
worthless. It's simply not true.
There's an excellent book available called *What Colour is
Your Parachute?* by Richard Bolles,[9] which is a practical guide
on how to re-enter the workforce. This book will help you
to determine what skills you have acquired and how they
can best be put to use (in other words, what type of job you
are best suited for). It also gives suggestions about how to
go looking for a job, how to prepare your resumé and how
to handle interviews.
Job hunting isn't easy for anyone, but try not to be
discouraged too easily. If a job is what you want, go for it!
(And don't forget about skills you may have learned as a
voluntary worker for organizations.) By the same token, if
you want to become involved in voluntary work, make sure
you get something in return—like skills you can use as a
stepping stone for a paid job.

Our role with partners

If we don't have activities which can cushion the lifestyle change which occurs when our children leave home, we may have to face a situation in which our relationship (or lack of relationship) with our partners is thrown into sharper focus. It may coincide with a time when our partners are also facing the prospect of retirement and are having totally to rethink their lives. It may also be that our partner is at the very peak of his career and is totally wrapped up in that. Or it may be that he is facing a lot of competition from younger men or has to face the fact that he won't ever achieve the positions he would like to. And because, statistically, men of this age are in a high-risk death rate area, it may be that some of us will be faced with the loss of our partner at the same time as we go through menopause.

One of the paradoxes of our society is that while women supposedly become less 'marketable' as they get older, men supposedly become more so. This is a time, then, when some men go looking for younger partners. While that's seen as acceptable in society, it's still relatively unacceptable for *us* to go looking for younger male partners.

All of these situations add up to extra stress for us at a time when our lives are undergoing major changes anyway. Again, as in all the periods of major upheaval, our relationships might need a major overhaul, or just a minor one. This can be a painful process, but it can also have satisfying payoffs. It may involve issues as big as 'Do we stay together?', or it may involve a complete reassessment of the roles each of us plays in relationship to one another.

You might find that in the past you've been playing out fairly rigid roles, with you doing certain things and your partner doing others and neither of you particularly enjoying doing what you think you have to. No relationship is static, and it can be changed if it's not as satisfying as it could be.

Some women who come to our courses have spent considerable time sorting out new marital arrangements and responsibilities. Some of the issues they've looked at include:

- Can housework—cooking, cleaning, shopping, laundry —be shared?

34

- What are the financial arrangements of the partnership? Do you have any say in how the income and expenses are divided?
- Transportation arrangements—do you share the use of the car (if you have one)?
- Do you need to reorganize your living arrangements? Are you happy about where you live? Do you have a room to yourself where you can be on your own? Would you like separate bedrooms?
- Do you have personal freedom? Are you able to get out with other friends without having to explain yourself? Can you take up separate interests from your partner?

Some of the women had come to other arrangements, such as agreeing on nights of the week which they could spend with other friends, and taking total care of the housework on alternating days.

Ageing parents
For many of us, menopause happens to coincide with a time when our parents, now old, need us to look after them. This reversal of roles—with parents looking to their children for care and support, rather than vice versa—can be upsetting for many women. So can the emotional and physical load of dependent parents. Decisions on whether our parents might have to be looked after in rest homes, the nagging stress of possible serious illness or death, the difficulty of balancing the various demands of our own children, partners and parents against our own needs can cause a lot of distress.

Recognition helps
Recognition of the things which are happening to us can help us to feel more 'in control' of our lives. To air our feelings is also important. For most of our lives we've been taught to keep the lid on our emotions. We've been taught to be 'copers', and we fear the labels of 'whiner' or 'nagger'. But like the proverbial sweeping of dirt under the carpet, sooner or later we've got to do something about letting feelings out. There's nothing wrong with that.

'Having no-one to confide in' is one of the four most strongly predicted reasons for depression. And over and

over again the women in our sessions have said they've felt
'immense relief' at being able to talk to one another:

> To find out that I wasn't going mad was wonderful—to find out
> that it wasn't just *me*—that I wasn't alone.

After seeing over 2000 women going through our sessions,
all of us involved with them feel very strongly that sharing
information and feelings is one of the most beneficial things
that women—of all ages—can do. To be able to feel that we
can do something to help ourselves is important, and to be
able to talk, compare experiences and see that the problems
which we think are exclusive to us are shared by many
others is one of the best ways of helping ourselves. We may
not be able to change the way society sees us as older
women, but *we* don't have to accept and believe the
stereotypes. I include details in Chapter 11 on how to set up
your own menopause group or discussion group.

How long will it last?

One point worth stressing after all this is that menopause is
not a permanent state of affairs. The things which might be
worrying you now could end as suddenly as they started.
And when the transition has been made, many women
report increased vigour and enjoyment of a life of PMZ—or
post-menopausal zest, as it's called.

'If you suffer from pre-menstrual tension, you can now
anticipate its demise,' said one woman jubilantly.

The transition can last from only a month or two to a few
years. Here's how a few women who have stopped having
any symptoms and now consider themselves to have
finished menopause look back on their experiences:

> Mine lasted about five years. I have aged, of course, but so has
> my husband. I think we are better friends than we used to be.

> Now I've finished I feel much fitter, sleep better and feel
> happier within myself and in the company of others. Sexually
> there is now much more enjoyment. I am more assertive and
> depend more on my own strength than on others. I am also
> better organized to cope with down days.

> From start to finish, my menopause lasted eight years. I've
> found a new freedom in all areas.

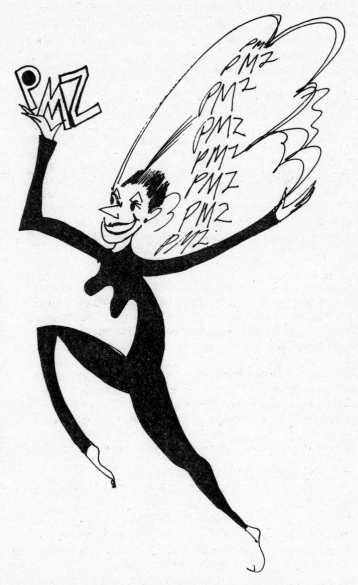

Many women report increased vigour and enjoyment of life after menopause. It's often called post menopausal zest.

Mine lasted about three years—it's hard for me to say.

I've been going through menopause for about 12 years and I still get light hot flushes from time to time. My mind is still a bit muddled at times and I'd still rather catch the bus than take the car, but I can tell I'm nearly over it. I'm nearly my old light-hearted self again. I call myself retired and just do housework when I feel like it. Emotionally I'm very stable. Sexually I've slowed down a bit, but I like it that way.

Mine lasted about two years. Physically I feel fine and emotionally I feel really well. No more hassles with nappies or flooding. Sexually there is a difference as I have noticed a significant drying up of my vagina.

I started having the first symptoms of menopause about 1976 and haven't had a period since 1979. Physically I now get tired easily but after a short rest feel better. I lack energy but after a short rest I'm all right. If I do feel a down day coming on I can cope better.

Mine took nine to ten years. Physically I feel older—I am arthritic. But in my whole life situation I feel as though I've had a rebirth. I may be in my later years but I'm going to make the most of them. I feel as though I have serene calmness and I now behave as I want to not as I think other people think I should.

Two books of relevance to jobs and health at this time are *A Woman's Work Book*,[10] and *Our Bodies Ourselves*.[11]

FOUR

The Medical Options

> About the time when the change is to happen—or not long after—many persons find the disorders to which they have heretofore been subject, more frequent and more troublesome. Some are afflicted with the well-known symptoms of plethora, heat, flushings, restless nights, troublesome dreams and unequal spirits.[12]

The effects of menopause have been surprisingly well documented down the centuries—and the symptoms noted even in 1750 (above) are still the same as those reported today. In fact, although we have a greater knowledge of how the hormonal system works than our forebears did, we're not a long way further down the road in our understanding of why some of the symptoms occur around menopause. We do know more about the specific effects of decreased oestrogen on our bodies, but we know little more about the way hormones affect our moods and feelings.

Many of the recorded studies show considerable empathy with women experiencing the effects of menopause. But some doctors had some alarming and bizarre views. Dr Anna M. Galbraith said in 1904[13] that in her view the menopause indicated some changes 'which started reasonably and mildly as loss of interest in daily affairs of life' but which quickly advanced to the stage of 'melancholia, insanity (delirium, mania, hypochondriasis), irresponsible impulses and—eventually—perversion of moral instincts'. With that rather alarming summary of events she concluded that it would be unwise for a woman to marry during menopause. Frankly, it's hard to imagine how any woman would have had the time and energy even to think of marriage if she was suffering from all the ailments which Dr Galbraith had diagnosed!

And there were other warnings, too:

> Perhaps the most common, and I really think the most terrible form of mental disease which is developed at the climacteric, is

the tendency to abuse alcohol . . . but by far the larger number of these unfortunates have adopted the habit late in life as a relief from their climacteric discomfort. These are the cases of insanity and it would be a wise law which would enable us to place them in seclusion till the time of trial was over.[14]

However, if the prognosis was alarming, so too were some of the cures. Blood-letting was most in vogue and worked on the theory that if you took away the blood, other injurious substances would be drawn off at the same time. It was assumed that because women going through the menopause were no longer bleeding, the blood must surely be accumulating in the system. The most common method of blood-letting was to place leeches on various strategic parts of the body and let them get on with their work.

Purgatives—'full doses of opening medicines'—were also heartily recommended for most symptoms. In 1889 one researcher wrote enthusiastically:

For the relief of nearly all subjective symptoms of the climacteric period I know nothing better than the use of an occasional purgative and removal from home at frequent intervals . . .[15]

Some of the more benign treatments included baths of various sorts and trips to the sanatorium. Some of the less benign were mixtures which included bromide, mercury, diluted sulphuric acid (for excessive bleeding from 'the female passage') mixed with lavender or cinnamon to make it more palatable, belladonna (or deadly nightshade, as we more commonly know it) and pills of acetate of lead.

The taking of opium was also warmly recommended, and one editor added a footnote to a research article noting that it had been 'accidentally discovered that Indian Hemp taken as a tincture, three times daily, could restrain uterine haemorrhage with considerable success'.[16] Indian hemp is, of course, marijuana.

But interestingly enough, some of the medical researchers hit on hormonal cures long before they realized how the hormonal system worked. Herbalists recommended pulsatilla and sarsaparilla—the former, at least, is known to contain hormones. In 1908, one researcher said that varying results had been achieved with various gland extracts—thyroid, ovarian and parotid. And the administration of dried corpus luteum from a pregnant animal, usually a pig, had been followed by a 'great improvement' in patients.[17] Earlier, a report in the *British Medical Journal* in April 1897[18] had claimed great success in curing flushings using ovarian extracts. (Not surprisingly, the same doctor had found that his other treatments—one of which was arsenic—had not been successful.) And in another bizarre forerunner to hormone treatments, a Frenchman, Charles Edouard Brown-Séquard, tried giving women two sheep's ovaries a day sandwiched between slices of unleavened bread. When this didn't work, he prepared extracts from the ovaries taken from mares, sheep and cows at their most sexually active age.[19] This suggestion stays in the history books for its novelty value rather than its success . . .

But what treatments do the 1980s have to offer?

Hormone treatment is, of course, the one that has received most publicity over the last 20 years. It's known variously as ORT or ERT (oestrogen replacement therapy, depending on how you spell oestrogen) or HRT (hormone replacement therapy). However, its acceptance hasn't all been plain sailing.

Some years ago, in a great flurry of excitement, oestrogen therapy was being hailed as a treatment which could make women look young forever. One American doctor, Robert Wilson, was responsible for most of this push for oestrogen. Women from all around the world flocked for treatment after reading his book—though it was in the United States that its popularity was particularly strong. It took the medical profession some time to counter the claim. Even now the belief that oestrogen treatment equals youthful looks still surfaces in our groups, and some drug companies still hint that it is a benefit of oestrogen therapy. Serious researchers refute this absolutely, and those who suggest that oestrogen therapy is a recipe for youthfulness are doing women a real disservice.

An equally serious claim was that oestrogen treatment was the answer to *all* menopausal problems. This, too, is quite incorrect.

In the past, oestrogen treatment consisted of large continuous dosages. What this did was to keep building up the lining of the uterus so that it was not sloughed away as in normal periods. Following these treatments, it was found that administered oestrogen was linked with a cancer which occurred in the lining of the uterus (endometrial cancer). Subsequently, the medical profession hesitated to use the treatment at all. Now, however, with the adjustments to a much lower dose of oestrogen and the addition of progestogen (the artificially produced equivalent of progesterone), the therapy is being used again—with much more care.

The theory—very simply—behind oestrogen treatment is that the administration of small doses of oestrogen helps to smooth out the surges and dips in hormone production that are sometimes experienced as we go through the transition. These surges are caused by one part of our hormonal system prodding another in the chain in an attempt to re-establish the hormonal pattern we've had since puberty. Oestrogen treatment, however, helps only a few of the effects of menopause. Professor John Hutton, a specialist in menopause research, says that he has had some success in preventing hot flushes and sweats and in halting vaginal dryness by using oestrogen treatment. And he says, cautiously, that oestrogen treatment may also help some cases of osteoporosis. But it is *not*, he says emphatically, a universal cure-all.

Oestrogen, with progestogen, is now given cyclically, thereby imitating our own hormonal cycles before menstruation stops. For about 21 to 23 days of the month you take a low dose of oestrogen; for the last seven to ten days of the treatment you take progestogen as well, and when both of these are stopped and if the lining has built up, you will bleed—as in a period. As the symptoms disappear with time, the treatment is gradually decreased and eventually stopped—usually after about a year (unless you are being treated for osteoporosis, in which case you may have to stay on the treatment indefinitely, since bone loss will begin again once the therapy has stopped).

If one of the things you like about menopause is the fact that you no longer have periods, the return of bleeds which resemble periods may be a drawback of this treatment. You may also not like the idea of taking hormones. Some of the pros and cons of oestrogen treatment are discussed by Vidal S. Clay in *Women,*

Menopause and Middle Age, and these are worth reading, despite the fact that the book was published in 1977 and bases its information on the high-dose treatments given until a few years ago. Two research papers which may be helpful to you or your doctor have also been published recently by Professor Hutton, the first giving a full description of treatments and dosages, and the second being an update on this information.[20]

Some notes of caution:

Sometimes oestrogen creams are prescribed for dryness of the vagina or for infections caused by that dryness. It's important to know that because oestrogen is absorbed through the lining of the vagina, it should be monitored *extremely* carefully, and the quantity of cream used kept to a minimum.

Some women tell us that they are still being prescribed a type of pill which contains androgens (male hormones) as well as oestrogen. The androgens in this hormonal cocktail can cause heavy hair growth in women. No woman, says Professor Hutton, needs to take androgens during menopause.

Some women cannot have oestrogen treatment. It is unsuitable for those who have shown a predisposition to diseases such as cancer of the breast or endometrium, and women with high blood pressure or heart problems usually can't be treated with it either.

For those unable or who don't want to take oestrogen, other non-hormonal treatments which are sometimes prescribed are:

- *Dixarit:* For mild hot flushes and headaches of which the primary cause is thought to be the flushes.
- *KY Jelly:* For vaginal dryness. This jelly can be bought from a chemist without prescription.
- *Tranquillizers, antidepressants (which are given to 'lift' depression) and sleeping tablets:* Some women who have come to our sessions have said that they felt angry and resentful when given tranquillizers and antidepressants. They felt that their doctors were merely fobbing them off rather than trying to get to the root causes of their depression. Others have said that they've been grateful for the option of using them when going through a bad patch

and needing a prop to enable them to cope. Sometimes antidepressants can help temporarily, but they don't help the *physical* symptoms of menopause.

- *Vitamins:* Some women say that vitamins have helped them during menopause. This is discussed in more detail in Chapter 7.

If you find it hard to talk to your doctor but want specific information on any particular form of treatment he or she prescribes, make a list of all the things you want to ask before you go. If you think you are not getting sympathetic or thorough enough treatment, you *can* change to another doctor.

Menopause and hysterectomy

Two questions which come up frequently in our sessions are:

1 'If I have a hysterectomy, will I still go through menopause?'
2 'If I have a hysterectomy, does it mean I'll have an early menopause?'

The answer to the first question is yes, since the only thing which has been removed in a hysterectomy is your uterus, and not your ovaries. However, you won't experience one of the visible signs of menopause—changes in your periods.

The second question is interesting. Many books say that if you have a hysterectomy and providing you have some ovarian tissue left, you will go through menopause at the normal time. Not infrequently, however, women have told us that they have experienced typical menopause symptoms such as hot flushes shortly after a hysterectomy.

Professor Hutton agrees that this can happen, and he puts forward several possible explanations:

'Hysterectomy is not a minor operation—it's a major one. It can be stressful and we know that stress can stop women having periods. Ovaries can also be affected, and if that happens women can get menopausal symptoms. If it is stress, it should come right and symptoms should disappear.'

A second possible reason for the occurrence of symptoms after a hysterectomy is that the blood supply to the ovaries may be affected in the operation, either through scarring as the area heals, or because the ovaries have been drawn down in the operation and the blood supply cut off. In these cases, too, your system should eventually return to normal.

In some cases, though, the reason for undergoing a hysterectomy might initially have been connected with some disorder of the ovaries. 'Although the ovaries may look normal when you look at them during the operation, their function might in fact be already impaired. These women might run into trouble later on,' says Professor Hutton.

One further recent theory is that the functioning of the ovaries may depend upon the total complement of follicles —or egg cells—left after surgery if one or part of an ovary has had to be removed. 'If you remove, say, one ovary, then you may cut down the chances of ovulation in the other ovary,' says Professor Hutton. 'The old premise of "Well, you've still got one left, you'll be fine" may not necessarily be true. You will have some ovarian function, but it may not be quite adequate.'

Medical help can alleviate some of the problems of menopause, but many women don't need or want medical advice. Often all we need is to know what's happening to us and to receive some support and understanding from the people around us. More on this in Chapter 11.

FIVE

Contraception

Much is made about 'change of life' babies. But the reason
we do hear about them when they happen is that they are
relatively rare.

The Guinness Book of Records records the birth of a daughter
to an American woman who was 57 years 129 days old. And
two women in Britain dispute the UK title—one woman
having had a tenth daughter at the age of either 54 or 55
years three days, and the other woman having had a son at a
definite 54 years 40 days.[21] (The Irish, slightly ahead in this
particular competition, reliably recorded a birth to a woman
55 years 69 days on 17 March 1931.)

Birth-rates and abortion-rates in the menopausal group
tend to be very low. The reason for the low incidence of
conception is that by the time we reach our mid-40s, our
egg cells have dwindled and those which are left are of fairly
low quality because of their age. They are therefore often
not capable of being fertilized. But statistics are one thing,
reality another, and for those of us who don't want to have
children at this age the possibility of pregnancy can be
frightening. We know that the chances of our giving birth
to Down's syndrome (mongoloid) children are greatly
increased after the age of 40, and we are told that the risks
from haemorrhage and problems with blood pressure and
kidney functions are also increased after 40. Those are risks
few of us are prepared to take.

There are many differing views on when it's safe for us to
stop using contraception once we have stopped menstruating. Some doctors say that contraception should be
used for a year after our last period. Most doctors now
advise women over 50 to continue with contraception for a
year after their last period and women under 50 to use
contraception for two years after their last period.

Methods of contraception, in brief

The following is a brief rundown on the various methods of contraception. Most of these methods will be quite familiar, but it's worth reminding ourselves of the choices from time to time.

Oral contraceptives

There are two kinds of oral contraceptive. The combined pill contains varying proportions of the hormones oestrogen and progestogen and works by suppressing ovulation. It also affects the lining of the womb so it will not receive a fertilized egg, changes the consistency of the cervical mucus and alters the movement of the Fallopian tubes to slow the egg's passage. The second type, the progestogen-only (or mini) pill works by the latter three ways.

Injection

Depo-Provera contains only progestogen. It works in a similar way to the mini pill, given every 12 weeks and is a long-term method of contraception for women unable to use any other type.

Noristerat, given every 8 weeks, is for short-term use by women whose partners have had a vasectomy and are awaiting sperm clearance, and for women immunized against rubella during the virus' active period.

IUCDs

Most are plastic and copper devices (the Lippes Loop is entirely plastic) about 3 to 4 centimetres in length. These devices are inserted into the uterus and it is thought that they prevent implantation of the ovum by altering the actual lining of the uterus to a small degree. The copper is thought to prevent fertilization.

Barriers

Condoms, diaphragms and various caps are all used with spermicides. As their name suggests, these work by stopping the sperm from meeting the ovum. The contraceptive sponge is a new device that is impregnated with spermicide.

Spermicides
Not recommended on their own, but nevertheless better than nothing. They act as a chemical barrier between the sperm and the ovum. Foam is probably preferable to jelly or cream.

Which form is best for us at this age? Generally speaking, we can carry on with the method of contraception we have always used, providing that it has always been acceptable and problem-free.

However, if you are on combined oral contraception, and either smoke or have a family history of hypertension or coronary artery disease, it is advisable to change to another method as the risks of a stroke, heart attack and/or serious blood clotting are much higher than average once you pass the age of 35. A woman can use the combined pill until the age of 45 in the absence of any medical problem. It is difficult to know when a woman on combined oral contraceptives has reached menopause, and this necessitates her using another method while waiting to see if she is still menstruating.

The progrestogen-only pill is often a useful form of contraception at this age because it does not disguise the end of menstruation. But, like most things, it has both drawbacks and advantages for some people. You may have irregular bleeding or spotting and, very occasionally, heavy bleeding. Blood pressure may be slightly higher than the norm on the mini pill. Depo-Provera also comes into this category but its action is a bit different in that periods cease and again, dosage has to be stopped to see if periods return. Unless there are other reasons, such as the loss of a partner, which render its use unnecessary, doctors usually maintain Depo-Provera injections until the age of 48 to 50, when the risks of pregnancy are minimal.

Much controversy surrounds the use of Depo-Provera with claims that it may cause cancer. It can also cause unpredictable bleeding patterns and sometimes depression. Some women put on weight while using Depo-Provera and although probably not a particular problem at menopause, it may take up to a year for fertility to return in some women.

Barrier methods and spermicides are very useful at this age and have many advantages for menopausal women—not the least of which is the fact that they do not disguise the end of menstruation and usually have no physical side-effects. If your pelvic muscles are in good order, you can safely use a *properly fitted* diaphragm and a spermicide. Alternatives are small caps that work by suction, and the arcing spring diaphragm. A weight change of more than 3 kg, a miscarriage, abortion, or childbirth can alter the correct fit of the diaphragm and reduce its safety. You should have it checked every six months. Some women, too, are allergic to the rubber of a diaphragm or to the spermicide.

Cervical or vault caps can be used for those with poor muscle tone, and again must be used with a spermicide.

Condoms have been around a long time, and the current selection—which comes in various weights and colours—is a far cry from the bits of sheep's gut which were used over two centuries ago. Condoms have an additional bonus in that they reduce infection, pelvic inflammatory disease (PID) and some sexually transmitted diseases (STDs), as well as reducing the chance of getting cervical cancer.

Permanent methods of contraception

What of the permanent methods of contraception, such as tubal ligation, hysterectomy and vasectomy? Generally speaking, sterilization should only be considered if no more children are desired. It should never be carried out as a solution to contraceptive problems. All surgical procedures have risks, and should not be undertaken lightly. Admittedly, the risks are small in these cases, but the possibility of an unsuspected complication always exists. A hysterectomy may, of course, be necessary for women with gynaecological problems. In most cases of hysterectomy, only the uterus or womb is removed and the ovaries are left, causing infertility.

Tubal ligation is the simple division of the Fallopian tubes which allow the passage of the egg to the uterus. All other structures are left intact, so a woman may still need a hysterectomy several years later if problems arise.

The procedure for female sterilization

The first step is to obtain a referral from your doctor or the family planning clinic to the hospital in your area, where social and medical indications for sterilization will be assessed. There may be waiting lists for this operation, sometimes longer than six months. The public hospital may ask your partner to give his consent for the operation, although this is not a legal requirement.

If you request a referral to a private hospital or non-profit making charity, it is for you and the specialist to come to an arrangement about the time and the cost of the operation.

Vasectomies

Quite a straightforward operation from a procedural point of view, vasectomies are increasingly common. As for tubal ligations, the man starts with a visit either to his general practitioner or to a family planning clinic. He is then referred to a specialist, another general practitioner who specializes in doing vasectomies, or sometimes to a hospital outpatient department. Some surgeons require the consent of the patient's wife, but that's not a legal requirement.

Abortion

Abortion is not a contraceptive measure. However, if you think you may be pregnant and want to seek an abortion, then you should not wait too long. Dangers increase as the pregnancy develops and so the danger of the procedure will weigh against the benefit to the mother.

The following steps need to be taken. Get a pregnancy test from your general practitioner, family planning clinic, or from a women's group, pregnancy charity, or local chemist. (Because of irregularities in menstruation around the time of the menopause, there could well be a chance that you're not pregnant anyway.)

If the pregnancy test is positive, you and the doctor must discuss the choices open to you. If the doctor concludes that the continuation of the pregnancy is inadvisable under the grounds laid down by the 1967 Abortion Act, you will be referred to an operating surgeon.

Most abortion agencies will have follow-up procedures. There is no statutory requirement for such treatment, which may or may not be covered by your family doctor. At some stage during this process you'll be given contraceptive information.

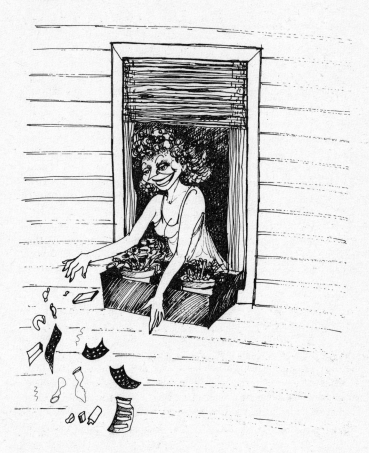

Being free of the worry of contraception and conception is one of the pluses of menopause.

SIX

Sexuality

Young people think they have a monopoly on sex. Well they don't. I've been sexual all my life and no one can tell me that suddenly, for some reason, I'm going to become a different person.

The links between menopause and sexual activity are hazy. Some women say they've never felt as positive about their sexuality as they have during menopause. Others, however, say that their sexual feelings and sexual activity wane at this time and many others say that they feel that this has less to do with menopause than with the state of their relationship with their partners.

In some cases, menopause does lead to tangible physical problems like heavy bleeding, vaginal dryness and bladder infections. Hot flushes and sweats and bloatedness also make life difficult for women who are feeling insecure anyway. As one woman said:

Not being able to rely on my own body made me feel sexually insecure, and for some time I withdrew from possible relationships because of this.

Our society feeds us messages about sex and middle age. The messages are that we have become sexually invisible. It's hard to put a finger on the age line which denotes sexual and non-sexual women, but one thing is certain—by the time we've reached middle age, we've supposedly crossed it:

I'm really worried that men will stop looking at me now. I'm scared that I'll suddenly have no sex appeal. I don't *feel* any less sexy, but it worries me that people will start treating me as though I *am* sexless. I felt that way about my parents—couldn't even imagine them having sex with each other—or anyone else.

So we become invisible, not because of any physical or other changes which happen to us but because society expects it of us. And sensing this expectation we sometimes

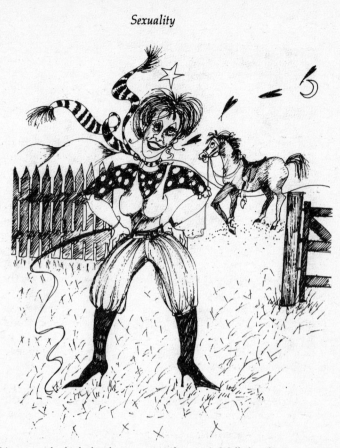

'Young people think they have a monopoly on sex. Well they don't. . . .'

try to hide or disguise our sexual needs, pretending that sex isn't of interest to us and feeling ashamed and embarrassed by our need for sexual contact and intimacy—a need basic to all people.

The truth of the matter is that we are all sexual beings and do have sexual and sensual needs. If we're no longer interested in sex it's usually because the right types of sexual relationships aren't available to us. Given the right conditions, the right partner, most women say they would want to be sexual.

Towards the end of menopause, many women experience a sort of rebirth, when their health is better than it has ever

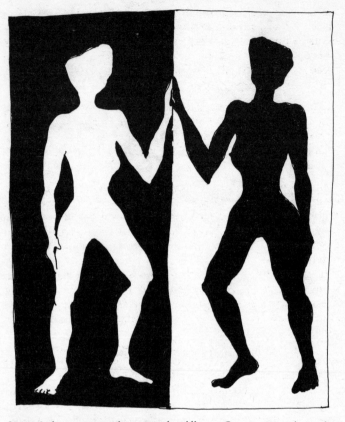

Society feeds us messages about sex and middle age. One message is that we have become sexually invisible.

been before, there is no longer the fear of conception and there are no demands from children to impede or thwart sexual pleasure: 'My feelings changed from something bordering on frigidity from fear of pregnancy to real enjoyment'. Sometimes, though, this rebirth—a nasty quirk of nature—comes at a time when our partners or other men of our age are suffering from their own sexual problems. For example, many older men find it difficult to achieve an erection—yet it is often we who take the blame for this, seeing our partners' frustration and problems as a reflection of our own lack of sexual desirability. Sometimes the male way of coping with such problems is to go off in search of a younger partner in the hope that his ebbing sexual ability will be restored. And even in relationships where this doesn't happen, the fear of partner infidelity still presents real difficulty for women at this time.

In her book *Female Cycles*, Paula Weideger says:[23]

> The common rationalization of such actions [men seeking younger partners] is that women are no longer interested in sex after menopause. This rationalization of course is presented in the form of a 'truth' and many women themselves come to believe it.

But there's a double standard. If *we* go looking for younger lovers at this age it's frowned upon. So while in theory we've reached a stage in our lives when we are more free to enjoy sexual relationships than ever before, in practice we're like the person who is all dressed up with nowhere to go.

It can be difficult for those of us without partners to know how to go about finding one. We have been taught that women are supposed to be passive if we want to be seen as 'feminine', but to be passive and wait for a partner to come to us doesn't work.

Women, like men, do have the option of masturbation— even though there seems to be a general assumption that men masturbate and women don't. Masturbation is neither better nor worse than other forms of sex. It is simply an alternative which can be enjoyed by all women—hetero-sexual or lesbian—in or out of partnerships. Certainly, there is an aura of guilt surrounding masturbation— something which has been overlaid with feelings of shame. But at least the subject is finally being brought out into the open, and though it may not be spoken about freely until our daughters' or even our granddaughters' generation, it is gradually being freed of such heavily loaded terms as self-abuse and self-pollution. Thank goodness.

Masturbation is a way of getting to know our bodies. It's a way of discovering what we enjoy sexually, what parts of us respond to what types of touching. And it's a way of discovering for ourselves what we want from a partner. Moreover, being able to masturbate to orgasm can take the heat off a partner to 'perform', and thus leaves both of you with more freedom to explore the sensual parts of the relationship.

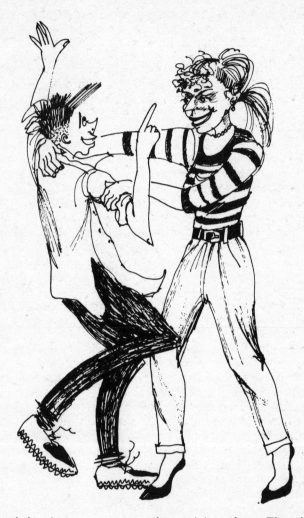

If we go looking for younger partners at this age it's frowned upon. They call it 'cradle snatching'.

Three women from our groups talked about their feelings on sexuality. Edith is 52. She and her husband separated two years ago after 25 years of marriage and two children, who are now independent adults.

> Now, two years later, I have a circle of men friends. Some of them are quite good friends but I don't feel ready for a long-term relationship. Perhaps that's because no one suitable has emerged, but I'm still optimistic.

Lorraine is 51, and has also separated from her husband.

> I was 39, in an apparently secure 22-year-old marriage, when it changed radically. For several years I went through valuable self-awareness groups. Now, after nine years of a financially secure single life, I feel independent and confident. At 51, I still sometimes yearn for the intimacy of being part of a couple and I'm still open to relationships, but I intend to enjoy the freedom of a single life. I've recently met a separated man and have developed a friendship with him.

Joan is 55. She has been happily married for 32 years. When her three children left home, she set up her own business, which she runs from her home.

> Although the last five years of our marriage has had its ups and downs, we are coming through that. Our sex life has changed but it's again close and satisfying.

The ideas and feeling expressed by these three women cannot, of course, be said to be wholly representative. Each of us has feelings and experiences which are unique to us alone. Their discussion, however, points to some of the major issues confronting women in menopause and demonstrates how the sharing of individual experience can be meaningful and reassuring for all those involved:

Raewyn We've talked about the way our culture sees us as middle-aged women. How do you feel this affects you?

Lorraine I feel it affects me because I do not see myself as a non-sexual person. I know very well that I am a sexual person, but I feel that the possibilities of relationships are limited because of the way other people see me. So it's a kind of on-going battle. I have to accept the changes in my life and my ageing, and work hard at being positive about these, because I feel that men and society generally see these in a negative way.

Edith I don't relate to this particular issue at all. I'm not attracted to men who are younger than me, so that may be the reason why it doesn't bother me personally. I am aware that many middle-aged men wouldn't be the least interested in women my age, but there are lots of men who aren't at all attracted to younger women. They are obviously the ones who attract me. I tend to think of those who care only about furthering relationships with younger women as silly and vain. The only time I feel I'm not a sexual person is when, for various reasons, I get into self-hatred and let myself go and put on weight. So, from time to time I feel like a nothing, but that's within me and has nothing to do with external influences. But I could be wrong.

Joan I feel that somehow I've got into a drawer that somebody's shut and that I'm no longer sexual. But it's nothing to do with society that I feel that way. I just don't feel like anything—let alone a sexual being. My menopause has gone on for so long I'm sure it has been compounded by a lot of things. I have shut down in every way and I'm no longer contributing sparkle to anything.

Lorraine When you don't feel good about yourself, then your sexuality does disappear, doesn't it? I think our attitude towards our sexuality is very much tied up with our feelings about ourselves as worthwhile people: our self-esteem. In order to feel sexual there has to be a certain excitement in the way you perceive yourself. I don't have very much in the way of relationships with men and my sexuality has diminished. But I feel that's purely because I'm not exposed to the stimulus. I still feel quite confident that the potential is there.

Raewyn One of the comments I picked up before was that given the chance everybody wants to feel sexual. Does that apply to you?

Joan Yes, that's the sparkle—the bubbles on top of the

glass. It needn't even be specifically sexual. If a man teases me then I start to bubble. It might have the promise of a relationship where sexuality might blossom. There are people, both men and women, who spark me off.

Edith   I define sexuality as a mental stimulus which, as you say, can be a woman-to-woman thing as well. Meeting any new person can be quite exciting, even though I have never been sexually attracted to a woman. A man is exciting to me because there's the promise of the physical thing. But it's still a mental thing, not purely physical.

Raewyn   A lot of people think of sexual needs in terms of straight sexual contact. When most women talk about sexual relationships they usually mean touching and getting and giving affection. Do you think your needs in a relationship have changed since you were younger?

Edith   I don't think my needs have changed very much at all, though I think I'm very much more aware of my own needs, rather than solely my mate's.

Lorraine   I still feel the need for closeness, for touching and intimacy and physical satisfaction, but that's the lesser part of it. The greater need is to be close to someone special. That's definitely missing from my life.

Raewyn   Having someone to care about you a lot?

Lorraine   Yes.

Edith   I agree with that. But the caring part has to be done by somebody who is interested in me and my thoughts. Even though some of my interests might appear somewhat extreme—politics and feminism for example—I can only have a worthwhile relationship with someone who is interested in me and who's definitely not patronising. It needs to be someone with something to contribute and who obviously doesn't think my interests are strange—some sort of disease that I'll grow out of sooner or later. I don't want someone to laugh at me or to say as some do, 'These women, such funny creatures.' This is a prevalent attitude.

Joan   What you are saying is you want someone to treat

59

you as a person. Not just a wife or a mother, but a person with ideas and opinions which need to be recognised as well as the physical patting which can or can not lead to bed, depending upon how you feel. It's part of being a complete person, not just someone who is physical, but someone thinking, too. I've been in a relationship for some 35 years and certain parts of it just slip away into the distance. Some parts have just not been listened to.

Lorraine That's one of the comforts for me, I guess. What appears to be very clear is that even the many people who are in partnerships, whether married or otherwise, are not getting their real needs for intimacy solved at all. Very many of my friends are discontented, and although I often yearn for closeness and intimacy with a special person, realistically I know it's not easy to attain. It's just fantasy or jolly hard work.

Joan The trouble is we all grew up on this fantasy of Happily Ever After. Nobody ever told us differently. It's a fairy tale somebody thought up. I don't think there's a Happily Ever After for most people.

Edith Well I still aim for that. I have certain criteria. I want somebody to be close and approachable, accepting on all levels. Someone who will hold my hand, who likes to cuddle and to be cuddled. So I seem to have a whole list of mental and physical requirements. I'm not prepared to settle for anything less—not at this stage. I don't think I'm being too demanding. I want someone who hasn't been horribly damaged in previous relationships. If they are so damaged they are not prepared to be vulnerable again, that's no good for me. It's a tall order, but I feel optimistic and think I may once again be involved in a long-term relationship.

Lorraine I think the thing you read about, use it or lose it, is very true and I feel sure even now that given a stimulating relationship my sexuality would blossom. But at present I feel my sexual needs are less. For instance, I masturbate a lot less than I did several years ago so my actual physical need is less. I also feel that an adjustment to a sexual relationship would now be quite hard because my body's different and I have to accept the limitations—dry vagina and thinning walls which are painful. I feel I could adjust to it—the potential is there, given the interest. Given the right partner too.

Joan   My husband's climacteric came about exactly the same time as my menopause and I went through a time wondering if there was somebody else, whether I was no longer attractive. It was hell for a couple of years. Now, if we miss this week . . . well, we miss sex this week. Before, if I'd missed sex even for two days I'd have been up the wall. So I've changed my demands. Whether this is because of the changes in my body or in my mental attitude, I'm not sure. I went through a stage when it was on my mind all the time. I had never had sexual fantasies, never looked at men in the street lustfully, but for two years I was a crotchwatcher extraordinaire. And I'd never before been interested in whether men would be all right to go to bed with. Life was too interesting and too full of other things. Then suddenly, just like when you intend to give up cigarettes, you can think of nothing else. When I was giving up sex and didn't want to, all I could think of was sex.

Raewyn   When was that and why?

Joan   Just before I started menopause, about ten years ago. I could have had sex three times a day, every day in the week had it been offered. Instead, I found myself living with a man who wasn't interested any more. We have had, and have again a very satisfying sexual relationship. It's close and it's satisfying. But suddenly, when he didn't want it, it was scary.

Even if he really wanted to mentally, it was physically an impossibility. That depressed him, and that in turn depressed me. We never really talked about it but I continued cuddling and teasing, kissing and chasing him, being no different from how I'd been for the many years before. I have always been a touching, loving person and I missed my children so much. Not having anybody to put my arm around, kiss, or to give a playful smack on the bum. My husband has never been demonstrative, and suddenly I didn't have the kids to share all this physical stuff with either. So this situation was compounded with my menopause.

Raewyn   Edith, you've recently separated from your husband. Did you find the same thing with him?

Edith   No, not really. Perhaps slightly less. I think he may have felt it more than I did because sex, for me, was a chore. It was awful and unexciting to say the least. I never really enjoyed it. He didn't seem to know about loving, sensual experiences that could go on for hours. Sex, for him, was only a tremendous orgasm, nothing else. I always felt insecure and upset. Always felt it was my fault. You can't be a yard apart mentally and suddenly come together in bed. I didn't know that then.

Looking back, it was a shame for both of us. A waste of all those years. It was scary, though, getting out of such a relationship. But once I had finished licking my wounds, I had to go about gathering men friends. I had no idea whether middle-aged men and women were promiscuous or not. So I made a big effort to get to know men. What I have found is that if at first I haven't been able to discuss the sexual side of a relationship, it's never going to get better. It's only looking back that I have realised it was awful. All the indirect messages I received about my lack of sexuality built up to a very big mountain. Although I didn't agree with this in my head, I didn't really know and I felt very insecure.

Raewyn   How old were you, Lorraine, when you and your husband separated?

Lorraine   Forty-three.

Raewyn   Have you had other relationships since?

Lorraine   Yes. I actually had others before we separated because we were into the open marriage thing. Originally I believed in a pair, didn't even consider having other relationships outside marriage and didn't think my husband would want to either. I was 39 when I found out that he wanted an open marriage. I guess I'm grateful now for the opportunity I have had. I found out a lot more about myself, even though it was a painful business. I would never have chosen it at the time because of my insecurity and dependence. Now I realise that it has been part of my growing, and the degree of confidence that I've got in myself is because I've now had lots of experiences. I had been protected from knowing that my husband had had extra-marital affairs and that a lot of men see this as perfectly acceptable and desirable. Had I continued to be protected I wouldn't have had the opportunity to grow and be aware in the way I am now. I feel I am more able to cope with aloneness and a single life because of the relationships I have had. I was very pleased when I did break up that I had the experimentation in the preceding four years. I feel if I'd been suddenly bereft of a partner from what had been a dependent relationship, I would have found it very much harder to cope.

Joan   At least you knew you were sexually attractive to other men.

Edith   It's very hard for the woman to be the initiator. If a man wants sex, it's so much easier as the passive partner to give. But if you want sex and he doesn't then it becomes a physical impossibility.

Joan   Mind you, I've found out that it needn't be. If you have a loving relationship, you can work on it and have sex. If you haven't got all those other things you say you want, then I don't think it will work. I have to be more active than when we were young. There are times, though, when I don't have an orgasm. I don't go along with the idea of going to endless lengths just to achieve an orgasm. I really don't, but perhaps I've been lucky.

Edith   Talking about orgasms, I don't have vaginal ones. It's an impossibility. I have never had an orgasm from intercourse.

Lorraine   Neither have I.

Edith   I think it would be absolutely marvellous to go through an experience detailed in a Harold Robbins book . . . where the earth moves. . . . Mine is a clitoral orgasm which doesn't happen with a penis. I can have an orgasm by using my hand. At one stage I felt inadequate about not having an orgasm during intercourse. When Shere Hite published her book it became clear that a large percentage of women don't have vaginal orgasms and I realised this wasn't peculiar to me. I'm surprised men don't know that most women are like this. I shouldn't have to spell it out. I feel that my partners should know that there are other ways of giving women pleasure.

Raewyn   He will have been brought up on Harold Robbins too!

Edith   Still, I expect a greater awareness. I enjoy sex anyway. It's the best form of communication I know. I feel it's very important that men are aware of the differences in women and are prepared to discuss them. It's nothing to be ashamed of.

Raewyn   Do you discuss it?

Edith   Yes I do, but if it's something they can't cope with then I'm put down and very disappointed.

Lorraine   I've got a lot of feelings about this because, like you, I have never had a vaginal orgasm and that seemed to me to be a big reason why, in our marriage, my husband became very enthusiastic about other women. I felt tremendously inadequate and would have been terribly comforted by reading *The Hite Report* many years earlier. A tremendous part of the experimentation that I went through was a desperate drive to learn how on earth I could have a vaginal orgasm. I felt it was my fault. During the experimental period I learned to be a lot less inhibited, but over and over again the male attitude was a puzzled: 'But when are you going to come? Don't you really?' It immediately became a challenge for them to try every bloody thing in the book from page 1 to 1001, to see if I would come. Either that, or they ended up feeling inadequate, dissatisfied and unhappy because they hadn't made me come. There doesn't seem to be the possibility of meeting an open man who accepts the way I am and the way I enjoy things and the fact that we're not going to have the great earth-shaking thing together with intercourse. It seems to me that this is part of my slight cynicism about future relationships.

Raewyn   If you have no really important relationship in your lives how do you cope with your sexual needs?

Edith   I've got a vibrator, which is very pleasurable. I don't know how often I use it, it varies. It's a physical release but a very lonely experience. I wouldn't like to think that it's all I have, but it certainly has its place.

Joan   Getting a vibrator seems a good idea. You do get into patterns of physical response, don't you? So by the time you're middle-aged and you've been doing it the same way for so long, it's hard to change initially. I didn't know I masturbated until just before my daughter married, when she came to stay with us and she mentioned the word. Suddenly the penny dropped. You are very lucky that you've had people you can talk to about sexuality because apart from one friend, I've never talked about sexual needs/drives with anybody else ever.

Raewyn   It really is a taboo subject isn't it?

Joan   It's a question of trusting other women and it's hard to find someone you can trust within a small community. They could go and talk about it, so you don't open up.

Edith   I've found the sharing with women infinitely better than discussion with any men I have ever known. The women in the C.R. group I was attending were people I really liked. They were good and positive, non-judgmental and had many interesting things to say. It was surprising that although we differed greatly in background, current situations and age, we had so much in common. I wouldn't like to think that I'd—in fact, I definitely wouldn't allow myself ever to get so involved in a relationship that I didn't have the time to meet and talk with other women. Looking back, the women in the group, as well as individual women friends, helped me to get over the loneliness and come to terms with the situation. For a while I thought I had a monopoly on misery.

Raewyn How do you cope with other needs such as affection, touching?

Lorraine Physically, I feel deprived. Emotionally I get as much as I can from a support system of friends. I know a couple who are there when needed. They are very loving and the wife doesn't see me as a threat so I can always go to them for closeness and real sharing. I appreciate that very much because I think it is rare for another couple to be so warm to a single woman. They only fill part of my need though. I have also found women friends great to share with, but I do feel deprived on a sensual level. I recently tried getting a nice massage which was enjoyable but expensive.

Raewyn So you really haven't found any solution?

Lorraine No. It's virtually just a matter of finding substitute emotional supports. That's what I look for. People who can give me some nourishment and acceptance.

Raewyn There's just one last question. You said you had made a big effort to widen your circle of friends. How did you go about doing this?

Edith After my marriage broke up, and it was very sudden, I tried to assess the situation, wondering how many men I knew. I knew none who weren't in partnerships and I was surprised to find that men whom I thought were friends of us both looked a bit embarrassed when I met them in the street. This upset me rather—another rejection. I realised I was a fool to think they had ever been friends—I was accepted as part of a couple, no more. I also realised that I was disadvantaged this way in that I worked solely with women. I thought I must let men know I exist. I went to some dances—there were some good single dances around. I didn't enjoy them though—felt I was too dependent upon a stranger as to whether I had an enjoyable evening or not. If I had only a few dances I got a bit depressed and I certainly didn't want to spend money and time in order to finish an evening feeling more miserable than when I'd started out. I did meet one man at a dance who was quite good company but it soon became obvious that he was in trouble with the police. This made me realise I wasn't likely to be introduced to someone whose background was known anyway. So I thought why not give the personal columns a try, stating my needs? I put an ad in, after going to a lot of trouble to get the wording right. I was amazed to receive a whole heap of replies and that made me truly aware there were many men around my age who were anxious to enter a relationship, or at least widen their circles of friends as I was. I think I put four ads in over the space of a year. I mentioned my actions to several friends who were all enthusiastic and helped make up ads and do some for themselves as well. We found it necessary to be cautious about humour. One ad a friend used was for a "sensual man", sensual being an awareness of all the senses, but that was mistaken and the replies were lecherous. Similarly, a reference to a "vibrant woman of middle years" conjured up visions of seething flesh. We quickly realised there was a happy medium and in order to get replies from people who were a little bit different I had to think up wording to attract a person with a bit of spark. The whole thing has been a lot of fun and a challenge. Making up an ad can be as much fun as meeting new people.

Raewyn   Where have you met them?

Edith   I have generally asked them home. I've not been entirely happy about that but I don't feel comfortable meeting them elsewhere. I have been a bit concerned about what my neighbours might think with different men calling on me, generally immediately after work. I think I have vaguely hoped they would assume I do a bit of typing.

Lorraine   I've had weird experiences with inviting people home so I don't do that any more.

Raewyn   Have you done anything similar to what we have just heard?

67

Lorraine Well, I guess I'm not quite that brave. I've tried everything but advertising. I've replied to ads which seemed a lot safer somehow. Perhaps taking the initiative is better. I've been to all the singles clubs around, starting off when I was alone as a solo parent. It was purely a social outlet for myself and that was about all there was in the early days when I was alone. I've tried the introduction bureaux, which are expensive, and only one long-term relationship came out of that. I suppose it's something. Another introduction bureau I tried was a real rip off. I think it's great you now have some men friends through your efforts. At this stage in my life I'd really like men friends who I could call up and suggest a visit to the pictures—male friends who are not necessarily expecting a sexual relationship. I have found so far with the men I've known that it's very much either/or. A relationship must include sex or there's nothing doing at all. I have found that the majority of those I replied to in the personal columns were just looking for a sexual relationship.

Edith One thing I *have* learned is that you don't find partners by sitting at home and waiting for them to come to you. I think it's essential for all women to join clubs—have lots of interests. The more things you're involved in the more chance there is of finding someone interesting.

Many of the women who have come to our menopause groups say that the sessions have provided them with their first real opportunity to discuss their sensual and sexual relationships and needs with other people. Many say that they've been really relieved to be able to talk in this way. Our sexuality *is* difficult to talk about, but because it is one of the most important areas of our lives it is also vital that it be brought out into the open—where it belongs.

An excellent book for woman of all ages which puts this topic into perspective is *Sex for Women (Who Want to have Fun and Loving Relationships with Equals)*.[24]

SEVEN

Food for Thought

Nutrition is a field in which opinions range so widely that there seems to be almost no common ground between experts. At one end of the scale we have the advocates of vitamin megadoses. At the other end are those who say that anything goes as long as we eat a variety of foods and don't eat too much of any one thing.

Vitamins are under a great deal of scrutiny at the moment. Some women who have used them regularly during menopause say that vitamin B_6 (taken as part of a vitamin B complex) has helped them to overcome tiredness and irritability and has improved their feelings of general well-being. (There are also some studies which say that vitamin B_6 is also helpful in the treatment of pre-menstrual tension.) Vitamin E is also advocated by some women, who say that it has helped to reduce hot flushes. Many nutritionists, however, believe that if you're going to take vitamin supplements you run the risk of creating an even more imbalanced diet than you might have had otherwise. Many take the approach that if you want to increase your intake of any particular vitamin you are better to do it through food.

It's up to you to decide for yourself. Even after fairly extensive reading on the pros and cons of vitamin supplements I can't say for certain whether they work—although a useful book on the subjects is *Women and the Crisis in Sex Hormones*.[25]

One thing I have found in common among women coming to our courses is that their diets are haphazard and often inadequate. Once families leave home, many women, freed from constant 'demand feeding', start eating scratch meals. Problems such as fatigue, which is common at menopause, are exacerbated by sloppy eating. Many women also put on weight at menopause. This comes in part from eating the wrong food, and in part from lack of exercise. But, fat cells produce some oestrogen, and there are some theories which suggest that the 'middle-aged spread' which most of us experience is the body's natural form of self-defence, enabling us to make a smoother transition between higher and lower levels of oestrogen production. But that should not deter us from caring about what we eat. It's relatively easy to ensure that we eat adequately—and without making a major performance of—if we know which foods provide which vitamins, other nutrients and calories.

I asked a lecturer in nutrition, Maria Thomson, to write the following section on nutrition in menopause. She has contributed to family planning courses on menopause, and has experienced many of the symptoms herself. In addition to explaining the function of the different nutrients she has worked out a suggested meal plan. A chart stating the various nutrients which occur in different foods and a calorie counter (both originally compiled by Dr John Swindells, a former Senior Lecturer in Nutrition) is included as well. These should help you to work out a diet suited to your own needs.

Diet and nutrition during menopause

For too long the subject of nutrition during menopause has been surrounded by a conspiracy of almost complete silence. Apart from the statement that calcium is lost at a considerable rate from the bones from the onset of menopause and that little can be done to stop it, no further mention is made in nutrition books of this very important period in our lives.

The various boards and committees which formulate dietary recommendations have ignored the menopause as a time of possible nutritional stress. No special recommendations to cover any additional needs that we may have as a result of altered body functions have been made. The statement that a 'normal' diet will cover all the needs of women at this particular age stems more from ignorance about nutritional requirements during menopause than from knowledge, because virtually no research has been done to find out if this assumption is correct. It is my belief that menopause affects our state of nutrition and that the alterations in the balance of a number of nutrients caused by hormonal imbalances may contribute to the symptoms of menopause. Some nutritional effects of menopause, such as the withdrawal of calcium from the bones, don't show up to their fullest extent until perhaps a decade later but are the results of a process which became a problem from the onset of menopause.

Before looking at specific menopausal symptoms which may be affected by nutritional factors, let's first consider whether your normal intake of nutrients corresponds to that which is usually recommended.

To give more meaning to this exercise, the following is a brief outline of the functions of individual nutrients and the foods in which they can be found.

Functions of nutrients

Together with nutrients which build the body and keep it going, we need vitamins and minerals to regulate and co-ordinate those body-building and energy-giving nutrients. There is, of course, a certain amount of overlap between functions. Protein, for example, serves both as a body-builder and as a nutrient essential for the formation of enzymes—the substances which bring about and regulate the many processes of our bodies.

Body-building foods

Protein. The word protein means 'first' and so implies that this nutrient is of major importance in nutrition. That is somewhat misleading, for *all* nutrients play a part in the economy of the body. It is true that without protein life is impossible, but we do seem to have overemphasized the role of protein in the past. Some of us actually eat more protein than is required for growth, for maintenance of the cells and for the manufacture of enzymes and hormones. A high intake of protein from animal sources may even lead to loss of calcium from the bones.

Calcium. Calcium is a component of our bones and teeth. It is the loss of calcium and other constituents from the bones which causes osteoporosis, discussed in previous chapters. Vitamin D, a fat-soluble vitamin developed in our skins by sunshine, helps the absorption of calcium and regulates the

71

laying down of calcium in our bones. Together with phosphorus, calcium gives our bones their strength.

In countries where the purdah is observed—that is, where women are compelled to cover their entire bodies, including their faces—and where the consumption of milk and cheese (rich sources of calcium) is low, many women have deformities of the bones, especially of the pelvis. Studies have also shown that the loss of calcium which causes brittleness of the bones in women going through menopause is seasonal; that is, it is more severe in winter than in summer. This indicates that the vitamin D manufactured by the rays of the sun moderates the severity of calcium loss and that women during and after menopause should ensure that they get some exposure to sunlight (vitamin D also occurs in fish-liver oils).

Many substances hinder the absorption and use of calcium by the body. A high intake of phosphorus through eating too much animal protein and cereals such as bran can have this effect.

Energy-producing foods

Carbohydrates. Starches and sugars are called carbohydrates. Starch is digested into glucose, which is metabolized to provide energy. Six of the vitamins of the B group are needed for the metabolism of carbohydrates.

The cane sugar we buy (its chemical name is sucrose) contains none of these B vitamins. We need to eat other foods rich in B-group vitamins to compensate for this lack. Another problem with sugar is that it is very quickly digested, giving the pancreas—the gland which makes insulin—a lot of work to do in a hurry. The insulin in turn acts by removing the sugar from our blood, thereby making us hungry again. This is no good for people who are watching their weight.

Fats. These are another source of energy—in this case, the stored energy from animals, nuts and some seeds. The main disadvantage of fats lies in the high number of calories they provide—twice as many as carbohydrates.

Vitamins

Fat-soluble vitamins. Fat-soluble vitamins apart from vitamin D include vitamins A, K and E. Few of us are likely to suffer from a deficiency of any of these vitamins: vitamin A occurs both in fatty dairy products and, in a less potent form, in highly coloured fruits and vegetables; vitamin K is available in adequate amounts in a balanced diet. Vitamin E is discussed in connection with hot flushes on p. 78.

Water-soluble vitamins. The main water-soluble vitamins are the B-group vitamins. The six which are needed to release the energy from carbohydrates are thiamine (vitamin B_1), riboflavin (B_2) niacin (B_3), pyridoxine (B_6) pantothenic acid and biotin. Other vitamins of the B group are folate and vitamin B_{12}. The inability to absorb vitamin B_{12} causes pernicious anaemia.

Folate or folic acid. Like vitamin B_{12}, folate or folic acid plays a part in the formation of cells. If insufficient folate is available to cover all the body's needs, the quality of the cells produced suffers. This can be seen readily in the mouth, where the gums become prone to inflammation, the tongue gets sore and ulcers may appear. The recommended allowance is 200 micrograms (µg) per day. Rich food sources of folate are liver, wheatgerm, orange juice, yeast and yeast products, and dark green vegetables. Long-term use of oral contraceptives will also deplete the body of folate.

Vitamin C. Beside protein, vitamin C is probably the nutrient of which people are most aware. The story of Captain Cook and his use of lime juice as a cure for scurvy amongst his ailing crews is common knowledge, and today vitamin C is widely advertised as a component of drinks and cordials.

Although it takes only 10 milligrams (mg) of vitamin C per day to cure scurvy, the recommended allowance is 50 mg per day. This not only provides a generous margin of safety but also takes into account the other functions of vitamin C in the body.

There are a number of scientists who say that we would be better able to resist all kinds of stress, including infection, if we consumed more vitamin C. They advise taking as much as 20 times the amount recommended as a daily intake, and some go even higher than that. Given that you would need to eat 10 to 20 oranges a day to achieve an intake of 1000 mg of vitamin C, those who think they might benefit from such a high intake will need to take it as a supplement, with medical supervision. However, because vitamin C and folate occur together in many foods, obtaining your recommended allowance of vitamin C from raw fruits and vegetables also boosts your intake of folate.

Iron. Iron is essential for the manufacture of red blood cells. Everyone knows that iron deficiency leads to anaemia. The reasons why this happens so commonly in women is because of blood loss during menstruation and the drain on iron during pregnancy. Women with heavy blood loss during menopause also need to ensure a good intake of iron.

Iron is a mineral which is difficult to absorb because it combines readily with other substances which make it insoluble. Vitamin C helps the absorption of iron and so does one of the amino acids found in meat and lactose (the sugar of milk).

Recommended allowances and sources of nutrients

The following is a brief summary of the most important nutrients, the amounts which are recommended as an adequate daily intake and some of the best food sources of them.

Protein. Adequate daily intake: 50 grams (g)
Best sources (per daily serving): milk (300 ml); meat, fish, liver (115 g); bread, cheese, egg (5–10 g); potato, nuts, legumes, green and root vegetables, gelatine, peanut butter (1–5 g).

Calcium Adequate daily intake: 600 mg
Best sources (per daily serving): milk, cheese (200–500 mg); molasses, ice cream, wholemeal bread, green and root vegetables, fish (40–100 mg); eggs, cream, white bread, oranges, meat, nuts, oatmeal (10–40 mg).

Iron. Adequate daily intake: 12 mg
Best sources (per daily serving): liver, black pudding (10–20 mg); wholemeal bread, kidney, meat (2–5 mg); green vegetables, molasses, eggs, white bread, nuts, fish, potato (1–2 mg); root vegetables, oatmeal, dried peas (0.5–1 mg)

Vitamin B1 (thiamine). Adequate daily intake: 1 mg
Best sources (per daily serving): pork chop, lamb's fry, bacon (0.4–0.6 mg); ham, wholemeal bread (0.2–0.4 mg); milk (300 ml), brains, mutton chop, green peas, Marmite, white bread, beef steak (0.1–0.2 mg); potato, wheatgerm, green and root vegetables (0.05–0.1 mg).

Vitamin B$_2$ (riboflavin). Adequate daily intake: 1.7 mg
Best sources (per daily serving): liver (3–5 mg); milk (300 ml), meat (0.2–0.5 mg); eggs, wholemeal bread, cheese, almonds (0.1–0.2 mg).

Vitamin B$_3$ (niacin). Adequate daily intake: 18 mg
Best sources (per daily serving): liver (more than 10 mg); meat, fish, kidney (6–10 mg); wholemeal bread, brown rice, peanut butter, peanuts, milk, white bread (2–6 mg); eggs, dried legumes, green and root vegetables, nuts, rice (1–2 mg).

Vitamin B$_6$ (pyridoxine) Adequate daily intake: 2 mg
Best sources: Although vitamin B$_6$ is very widespread in nature, few foods contain significant amounts—i.e., in more than 1 mg per 100 g. Meats average around 0.3 mg; wholemeal bread 0.18 mg; walnuts 0.73 mg; sunflower seeds 1.25 mg; bran flakes 1.38 mg; wheatgerm 0.65 mg and yeast flakes 2.5 mg. The last three items, however, are not usually eaten in 100 g quantities.

Vitamin C. Adequate daily intake: 50 mg
Best sources (per daily serving): blackcurrants (100–200 mg); oranges, kiwifruit, strawberries (50–100 mg); grapefruit, raw cauliflower, tomatoes, raw cabbage, gooseberries, grapefruit (20–30 mg); potato, swede, spinach, bananas, apples (10–20 mg).

Vitamin E. Adequate daily intake: 15 International Units (IU or mg)
Best sources: Being fat soluble, vitamin E occurs mainly in fatty foods, particularly oils from vegetable seeds. Margarine (made from oils) contains 8 mg per 100 g; butter 2 mg; wheatgerm oil more than 133 mg; whole egg 1.6 mg. Most meats contain only small amounts.

Folate. Adequate daily intake: 200 micrograms
Best sources: chicken liver (204 micrograms (µg) per 100 g);

brewer's yeast (313 per 1 tsp); spinach (164 per 1 cup); roasted peanuts (106 per 1 cup), beetroot (133 per 1 cup); almonds (136 per 1 cup); broccoli (101 per 1 cup); wheatgerm (118 per 30 g); orange juice (102 per 170 ml), liver (123 per 100 g).

Moderate sources: melon (82 per cup); parsnip (43 per 1 cup), frozen peas (37 per 1 cup); cashew nuts (95 per 1 cup). *Note:* 170 ml of orange juice daily will ensure that your minimum needs for folate are covered.

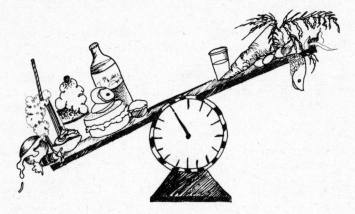

Does the food we eat affect the symptoms of menopause?

Withdrawal of calcium from the bones
According to nutritionists, there appears to be no convincing evidence that the taking of extra calcium makes a great deal of difference to calcium loss from the bones. However, I think we should at least make sure that we get enough calcium to cover the recommended daily allowance of 600 mg.

Milk and cheese are the main providers of calcium. They do have the disadvantage of being high in calories, but by choosing wisely we can minimize the risk of weight gain from these foods.

It's perhaps worth noting that while many nutritionists view the taking of extra calcium as futile, a group of women who were given 750 mg of calcium per day and 375 International Units (IU or mg) of vitamin D for three years showed no evidence of calcium loss. Please note, however, that under no circumstances should more than 400 IU of vitamin D be taken per day.

Whatever the pros and cons of calcium supplements may be, there seems to be no disagreement that regular physical exercise which puts stress on joints (such as brisk walking) helps to slow down the loss of calcium from the hip bones.

Weight gain and hot flushes

Although many factors contribute to weight gain, ultimately it is the greater input of energy in the form of food compared to the output of energy in the form of physical exercise which puts on weight—no matter how 'little' we may eat. This holds for men as well as for women. However, I have a hunch that the hormonal changes which occur at menopause affect our state of hunger or our need to eat. And it may be no coincidence that pregnant women and a number of people on oral contraceptives also put on weight.

In men, and women not going through menopause, sweating and palpitations which usually follow hot flushes can be caused by low blood sugar levels, or hypoglycaemia. This occurs before our contracting stomachs tell us that they are empty. Similarly, there may be a connection between hypoglycaemia and hot flushes (and weight gain) during menopause. This could explain the night sweats which often occur in the small hours of the morning when blood sugar levels are bound to be low because no food has been eaten for many hours. Eating to forestall this drop in blood sugar levels may help with hot flushes, but it is also likely to put on weight. It might therefore be a good idea to divide your total daily allowance of food into six small meals. By distributing your food intake more evenly throughout the day, the discomfort of hot flushes and the threat of unwanted weight gain could be minimized.

At the end of this chapter is a suggested outline of a day's eating plan. It can be used as a guide to organizing your food intake so that it is spread evenly throughout the day and does not exceed the total calorie limits recommended for weight maintenance.

Vitamin E as a means of alleviating hot flushes. Some women have claimed that vitamin E is helpful in reducing hot flushes, but no specific research has been carried out to confirm this. Various sources suggest, however, that a vitamin E supplement of 30 to 100 IU (mg) is sufficient to be of benefit. Vitamin E taken in excess of 100 mg is classed as a megadose, and a number of medical conditions may be caused by such high dosages.

Depression

Many of us seem to suffer from depression during menopause. As well as the external factors discussed in previous chapters, the depression associated with menopause may also have a biochemical or nutritional cause. Pyridoxine or vitamin B_6 has been shown to be a factor involved in many processes which affect not only the health of the body but also of the mind. It is used by some doctors and women's health groups to help treat the depression which is often experienced as part of the pre-menstrual syndrome. Many women who have attended menopause courses in different parts of the country also claim that they have felt brighter and livelier after taking pyridoxine. Vitamin B_6 seems to be inadequately supplied in the diets of many women.

Estimated normal requirements of vitamin B_6 are from 0.5 to 2 mg per day, but some experts consider that our requirements may be greater during pregnancy, in old age and if we use oral contraceptives. The dosage most often suggested is 25 mg, but most supplements contain 100 mg or more. Indeed, some recommendations seem to be ludicrously high—from 400 to 1500 mg per day. *I can't believe that there is any justification for the intake of any nutrient which is so much in excess of the normal amount used by the body.*

This statement also applies to multivitamin capsules and syrups. These may, in addition to supplying excessive amounts of specific vitamins (such as thiamine), also create an overall imbalance which is worse than no supplementation at all.

If you think that despite eating a 'good' diet you need to top off with food supplements, it is probably best to use only the specific nutrient likely to be lacking—for example, vitamin B_6 in moderate amounts and preparations such as liver tablets or yeast products—rather than expensive multivitamins. Both liver and yeast products are rich in vitamins of the B group and occur in an assortment which is more likely to meet the requirements of our bodies than are the products of drug companies. Some preparations of the milk powder-based type seem to contain a fairly balanced mix.

Lack of energy
Listlessness and a lack of vitality can result from low levels of vitamin B_6, as this can cause a type of anaemia which is not rectified by taking iron.

But as we have seen in previous chapters, there may also be a number of other factors involved, among them disturbed sleep patterns because of waking with hot flushes and sweats. While there's no easy solution to this kind of persistent tiredness, it is important not to allow your blood sugar level to get too low and to ensure that you get a liberal supply of essential nutrients as well as plenty of exercise, rest and relaxation. The suggested meal plan below may be of help here.

Suggested plan for six meals a day

Assuming that 1200 to 1400 calories per day are sufficient for a not very active middle-aged woman, each meal should provide only a little more than 200 calories. This means that you will have to choose your food carefully to stay inside the limit—and this can be done only by restricting your intake of sugar and fats. No more than 1 tbsp of margarine or butter per day is recommended, but make sure you include at least 300 ml of low-fat milk per day in your diet. Note, too, that meats, particularly beef, pork and mutton, are high in calories because of their fat content. Poultry (without skin) and fish are usually lower in calories, as are stews made with vegetables rather than meat alone. Depending on the kind eaten, meat will contribute between 150 and 400 calories per serving.

Breakfast
    Small bowl of muesli (homemade is better, and you can vary the ingredients) with low-fat milk

tea with low-fat milk (no sugar)
approximately 220 calories

Mid-morning
Small slice bread with 1 tbsp cottage cheese
1 apple or orange
tea with low-fat milk
approximately 140 calories

Lunch
Small piece meat (no more than 25 g), fish or low-fat cheese (i.e. Edam or Gouda), or egg
small slice bread with butter or margarine from daily allowance
medium salad made from any raw vegetables with low-calorie dressing
or
hearty vegetable soup made with fat-free stock to replace meat, with bread as above
170 ml glass orange juice (without added sugar)
approximately 210 calories

Mid-afternoon
Small slice bread with liver spread (here, too, homemade is better)
tea with low-fat milk (no sugar)
approximately 150 calories

Dinner
100 g lean meat
1 medium potato
generous helping green and root vegetables
1 piece fruit
approximately 440 calories

Supper
170 ml glass low-fat milk
1 water biscuit with slice low-fat cheese (Edam or Gouda)
approximately 150 calories

This adds up to approximately 1300 calories per day.

Some notes. A friend reading my notes has questioned the amount of bread I have suggested. Providing that the calories contributed by the bread stay within the overall limit, this amount is quite acceptable. However, homemade bread is fun to make, somewhat cheaper and more sustaining than commercial bread. A slice of homemade bread with Marmite or cottage cheese or just butter or margarine, a drink of milk or cup of soup and some raw fruit make a satisfying lunch.

All the suggested snacks contain protein, carbohydrates and a little fat. The protein and fat give your meal more staying power and keep your blood sugar on a more even level.

Remember that although you could eat a little more than suggested if you exercised, it takes pretty vigorous exercise to burn up even a small number of calories. For example, it takes 10 minutes of skipping to use up the calories from three sweet biscuits!

Desirable intakes of protective foods

Vitamin B-rich foods	at least three helpings per day
meat, fish, legumes, cheese, eggs or nuts	2–3 *small* servings per day
potatoes	preferably 1 per day; at least 4 per 5-day period.
all other vegetables and fruits	no less than 3 servings per day
orange juice (sugar free)	1 × 170 ml glass per day
other vitamin C and folate-rich foods	as often as possible
milk (low fat)	no less than 300 ml per day

The above notes on nutrition in menopause *may* help to eliminate some of the stress and discomfort associated with particular symptoms. But because each of us differs greatly in our experience of these symptoms, you should extract what seems most appropriate to your needs.

EIGHT

Stress

Stress is one of our biggest problems. How do we tell if we're under stress? What do we do about it? When I read down the list of symptoms which are reported by women coming through our groups, I can't help noticing the similarity between the symptoms of menopause and the symptoms that are commonly induced by stress.

Strain of any kind has a physical effect on our bodies. However, things that bother some people will not worry other people at all. What for some causes worry and anxiety, for others is an exciting challenge. It depends on our individual coping skills.

But first of all, what is stress? It's a word which is used a lot these days and has become quite fashionable. It has replaced words such as tension and strain, and is used interchangeably with anxiety.

Stress is the reaction of our bodies to the anxiety we feel when we are in a situation which frightens us or makes us feel uncomfortable. And as we have seen, these sources of stress vary from one person to another. As a child, visits to the dentist always made me feel really anxious—and they still do. On the higher end of the scale, falling out with friends or angry confrontations cause me great stress. Each of these situations is easily recognizable as stressful. On a day-to-day level, too, there are a number of things which can cause us stress. When I worked in a job I didn't particularly like, the thought, each morning, of having to go made me feel as though I wanted to be sick. Meeting new people or having someone for a meal when I'm not feeling very bright sometimes makes me feel the same way. Changing living arrangements, children leaving home, making an important phone call—each of these things can, to some degree or another, be stress-inducing.

The interesting thing, though, is that whatever the *source* of the anxiety, medical research indicates that our bodies react in a stereotyped way. The biochemical changes which

82

occur are identical and are essentially meant to cope with the increased demands which stress makes on our bodies.[26] The sorts of physical manifestations which have been recorded are wakefulness, trembling, palpitations, dizziness, muscular pain (knotted stomachs?), quickened heart beat, increased blood pressure and headaches. Sound familiar?

So, no matter what the cause of the stress may be, our bodies' reaction to the tension is standard. The first part of our body to react is the hypothalamus. Once this is stimulated, it sets off a complex chain of biochemical and neural processes, including the automatic nervous system which mobilizes our stress-coping mechanisms, and our pituitary gland. This releases a hormone into the blood stream which then stimulates the adrenal gland to release adrenaline and other biochemical substances. These further arouse the body's defence mechanisms. Our bodies are then in a state of preparation—for flight or fight. The heart beat increases, we breathe faster and deeper so that our bodies are provided with more oxygen and we perspire more. Our muscles tense ready for action, and the pupils of our eyes dilate. Actions such as digestion decrease. We are now prepared to fight or run if need be.

This is fine if we are in a situation which is going to demand one or other of these quick reactions. However, if we are constantly in a state of tension, our whole system starts to suffer from the wear and tear of trying to cope with this physical state of preparedness. Certainly our bodies try to adapt to this state of constant alarm, but in the process energy which would normally go into maintaining our other bodily processes is diverted. Gradually our bodies go into a state of exhaustion and our other physical functions can also break down.

Menopause can cause stress

We've already seen that many changes can and do happen around the same time as menopause. Anxiety, and especially anxiety about the direction of the rest of our lives, is the most often repeated area of concern for many of us. This is no small worry, and it would seem to be a pretty surefire recipe for high stress.

There is now a considerable amount of medical and

scientific evidence to link stress to physical and mental illness—ulcers and heart attacks are the ones we hear about most, but other illnesses such as arthritis and various allergic reactions have also been linked.

Two members of the University of Washington's School of Medicine, Thomas Holmes and Richard Rahe, have developed a questionnaire to look at the relationship between stressful events and illness. They also drew up a list of what they considered to be the highest stress-inducing events in our lives. These events ranged from the death of a spouse, divorce and marital separation at the top end of the scale to Christmas and minor violations of the law at the bottom end. Each event was given a certain number of points ranging from 100 to 11.

By marking the events which have happened to you in the previous year and by adding up the points given to each event, you then have a chance of seeing whether you are at risk of becoming ill. According to the authors' theories, if you score over 300 points you may well run the risk of developing a major illness in the next two years. If you score between 150 and 300, you may have a 50 per cent chance of a major health breakdown. A score of 150 or lower means a relatively low amount of life change.

Although this chart seems more slanted towards men than women, many of the situations can be reinterpreted so that they apply to our own lives. For example, retirement could mean our retirement from the role of mother when our children leave home.

From the list on page 85, check off each of the life events that has happened to you in the past year. Total the associated points and check your 'score' against the guidelines mentioned above. Remember, a score below 150 indicates a relatively low susceptibility to stress-induced health breakdown; a score of about 300 or over means that the odds on your experiencing a major health breakdown are about 80 per cent.

The Holmes-Rahe Life Stress Inventory[27]

Life event	Mean value
Death of spouse	100
Divorce	73
Marital separation from partner	65
Detention in jail or other institution	63
Death of a close family member	63
Major personal illness or injury	53
Marriage	50
Being fired at work	47
Marital reconciliation with partner	45
Retirement from work	45
Major change in the health or behaviour of a family member	44
Pregnancy	40
Sexual difficulties	39
Gaining a new family member (e.g. by birth, adoption, older dependant, etc.)	39
Major business readjustment (e.g., merger, reorganization, bankruptcy, etc.)	39
Major change in financial state	38
Death of a close friend	37
Changing to a different line of work	36
Major change in number of arguments with spouse (e.g., either more or less than usual regarding child-rearing, personal habits, etc.)	35
Taking on a large mortgage (e.g. purchasing a home, business, etc.)	31
Foreclosure on a mortgage or loan	30
Major change in responsibilities at work	29
Son or daughter leaving home (e.g., marriage, university, out-of-town job)	29
In-law troubles	29
Outstanding personal achievement	28
Spouse beginning or ceasing work outside the home	26
Beginning or ceasing formal schooling	26
Major change in living conditions (e.g., building new home,	

remodelling, decorating of home or neighbourhood)	25
Revision of personal habits (e.g., dress, manners, associations)	24
Troubles with boss	23
Major change in working hours or conditions	20
Change in residence	20
Change in school	20
Major change in usual type or amount of recreation	19
Major change in church activities (e.g., more or less)	19
Major change in social activities (e.g., clubs, movies, dancing, visiting, etc.)	18
Taking on a mortgage or loan of less than £10,000 (e.g. purchasing TV, car, freezer, etc.)	17
Major change in sleeping habits (e.g., more or less than usual, change in time of day or night)	16
Major change in number of family get-togethers	15
Major change in eating habits (e.g., more or less than usual, different meal hours or surroundings)	15
Vacation	13
Christmas	12
Minor violations of the law (e.g., traffic tickets)	11

How to deal with stress

The first step is to *recognize* the signs and to ask yourself honestly if there is some underlying worry which is making you feel physically ill or depressed. The next step is to identify those things which make you feel anxious. Note when they happen. Sometimes the reason may be easily apparent—like anxiety over marital separation, meeting new people or applying for a job—but sometimes there seems to be no apparent reason for anxiety, and all you can see are your own misery and feelings of helplessness.

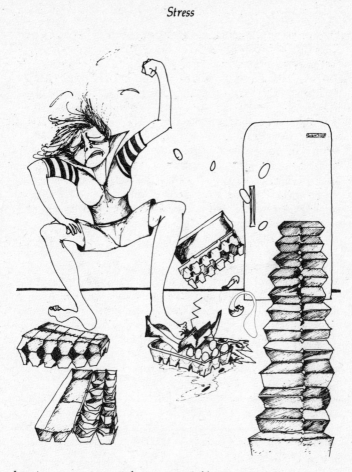

Jumping on egg cartons made one woman feel better . . . 'It helped me to feel less angry.'

It often *is* extremely difficult to work out what is at the root of our anxiety and there can be a number of contributing factors to complicate the picture. In Chapter 11 information is included on how to set up your own menopause discussion group. Don't be put off if the idea sounds a bit heavy. I've found groups such as these extremely worthwhile in helping me to analyse what it is that makes me feel the way I do. They also help you to get your own fears into perspective.

In some cases, though, talking with a professional counsellor may be the best means of coming to terms with anxiety and stress. This, too, can be threatening at first, for many of us are diffident about asking for help. We're scared that we'll be labelled as mentally ill or that a request for help will be seen as a sign of 'weakness'. We feel inadequate if we can't 'cope' with our own problems. If you feel like this about counselling, talk things over with a supportive friend. The counsellors whom I work with make the point that many people think that they have to be suffering from a 'real' crisis before they can go to seek help. They also make the point that the best time to sort things out is *before* a crisis occurs. You wouldn't wait until you had pneumonia before going to the doctor, would you?

Supposing that you feel you *can* handle what's happening to you alone, the first step is to look at what is worrying you as objectively as possible and then look at the way you respond to that situation. Do you feel you are over-reacting? Would you react the same way at other times? If not, why is it different this time? Ask someone you trust whether they think your response is appropriate.

The next step is to work out a plan of action to help yourself. Can you remove yourself from the source of stress? Are there things you like doing which would help you to feel better about other parts of your life and help to take the focus off the stressful things? We all have our own ways of making ourselves feel better.

At one recent menopause course I asked women what they did when they were feeling down. Here are some of the things they suggested:

> I've got this list of things I drew up one night of all the things I like to do or want to do but don't. When I'm down I go through the list and pick one of them to do. Some of those things are taking a train ride, going to the library, meeting friends for lunch.

> I'll go to the midnight movies and see if I can do it without looking over my shoulder to see who's watching.

> I go and get my feet done at the chiropodist.

> I decided one day that I would do something different. So I went out and got myself a motor cycle licence. I'd never even ridden a

two-wheeler! I thought perhaps I'd be too old, that I'd be the oldest person on the course and they'd all be 19 . . . I was, and they were. But I got it, and I really enjoyed having it.

To get rid of pent-up feelings and to avoid storing stress can be hard. A lot of women have said that they get benefit from taking long walks; another bought herself a dance record and dances 'furiously' to it. Another said that she found it very satisfying to 'save my egg cartons and jump on them when I'm angry'. Yet another, who had identified the source of her stress as her 'bone lazy son who expects me to run around after him like a slave', came up with another solution:

'I used to come home at night and find all his dishes still sitting in the sink, clothes on the floor. In the end I just put them all in his bed.'

Crying, too, is a way of releasing stress.

Longer-term solutions can range from the trite-sounding suggestion that you take a short holiday, away from the source of stress, to more dramatic moves like leaving your home and family. But in between there are usually a range of options, and many women find that learning such constructive coping skills as assertiveness training—that is, 'learning to stand on your own feet without standing on other people's toes'—is really helpful:

I went to an assertiveness group at a community house. Ten of us still meet once a fortnight. The result of it was that I wrote a letter to the paper about the rates—and I got it published! I thought, 'It's time I learned to look after myself'. I'm the granny of the group. We range in age from early 20s to my age (about 60). I've learnt how to approach personal problems, how to phase it right—to get what I want without pushing other people around. I feel as though I'm a person now, not a doormat for my family.

Assertiveness training courses are available in many areas, and quite a lot of books on the subject have been published recently. One of the best is called *Self Assertion for Women*.[28] It's full of excellent advice on how to deal with situations in which you feel you are being pushed to do what others want you to do rather than what *you* want to do. And we all know how stressful that kind of pressure can be.

Lastly, try and make a habit of doing some simple relaxation exercises. They do work and if you do them regularly you'll also find that you won't be getting as tense as you once did. Some people put the instructions on tape instead of having to memorize them.

1 Make yourself comfortable either in a chair or lying down.
2 Close your eyes.
3 Take in a slow, deep breath to the count of 10 and breathe right down into your stomach area, not just to your chest. Breathe out to the count of 10.
4 Continue breathing in and out to the count of 10 and think of a word which is peaceful to you. Repeat it each time you breathe out.
5 Tighten up the muscles in your right foot as you breathe in. Relax them as you breathe out. Repeat for your other foot, then for each leg, your buttocks, your stomach muscles, chest, each hand, arm, shoulders and neck.
6 Keep breathing rhythmically and check that none of your muscles have tensed up again. Stay sitting or lying like this for 10 minutes.

Do these exercises whenever you need to, but regard 10 to 20 minutes twice daily as indispensable!

NINE

Exercise

Disuse is the mortal enemy of the human body. We know today that how a person lives, not how long s/he lives, is responsible for many of the physical problems normally associated with advanced age.

The US Administration on Ageing sums up what many of us have begun to accept as fundamental to our enjoyment of life, not only in our most active years, but in our middle and later years as well. What else can I say about exercise that you don't already know? That you can save your life by exercising? That you can kill yourself by sitting around? The generalizations are valid enough. But one other important aspect of exercise is that it has been found to slow down bone loss and tends to keep the bones stronger. That's something that women in menopause should keep in mind.

It's up to you to choose the form of exercise which you find enjoyable and can manage most easily—although being enjoyable is probably the crux of the matter. There's nothing worse than trying to stick to an exercise regime you can't stand! Some of the women in our groups take up running, and that's probably the best form of exercise, both from a physical and a financial point of view. However, the number of horrified looks on the faces of those who don't run and who listen to the stories of those who do tell their own story. Yoga may be a more appropriate alternative for some.

If you do take up jogging, you may be interested in the following facts:

● Jogging conditions the lungs to process more air with less effort—oxygen is the key to the cardiovascular system.
● Jogging makes your heart—the most important muscle in your body—grow stronger, pump more blood with

each beat and reduce the number of beats by up to 30,000 per day.

● Jogging exercises the arms and legs and has a firming effect on muscle groups throughout your body, especially in your abdomen.

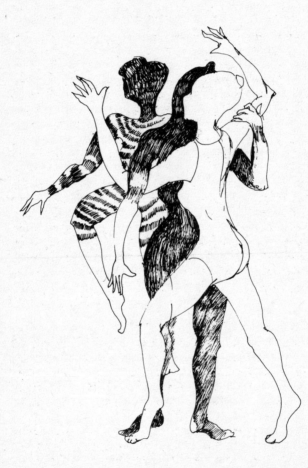

Exercise can be as diverse as you like. The important thing is to enjoy it.

All of those things play a part in improving our physical and mental well-being. However, the problem of how much or for how long a person should jog has bothered doctors and research workers throughout the world. Probably the best advice for beginners is to err on the side of caution. Any form of exercise done for any length of time is beneficial to some extent. Having tested your muscles, you should then gradually build up until you can maintain about 30 minutes of effort a day without straining. That doesn't mean fast jogging, it simply means jogging at whatever speed feels comfortable for you—mine is about fast walking pace. It's time on your feet that counts, not distance.

Another thing which often deters people from starting jogging (or any other 'public' form of exercise, like swimming or tennis) is the fear of *looking* exposed. When I first started jogging I felt extremely conspicuous. Now, I'm happy to say, there are so many joggers on the road no one looks twice. Everyone else is far too busy doing their own thing to notice. I run three times a week and only for about 20 minutes (or even less) each time. Even though that is regarded as a pretty low level of exercise, it's made a great difference to the way I feel, physically and psychologically.

Apart from the health benefits of women's running groups, they provide a good social life, too. You don't have to be 25, 8 stone (50 kg) and a former athletics champion to run with groups. They cater for people of all shapes, sizes and age groups.

Other types of exercise

Exercise can be as diverse as you like. It can range from active sports such as swimming and tramping to skipping, if you don't mind the boredom and prefer the privacy of your own home. In fact, some researchers say that skipping is probably one of *the* best ways of improving your cardio-vascular efficiency (getting fit).

Walking briskly is very good, too. One woman from our groups says that she makes a point of walking from her home to wherever she wants to go then catches the bus back. That way she doesn't have to look at the same scenery, either! Another woman has said that not only had her health benefited from walking, but her garden had also flourished, thanks to the huge variety of cuttings she'd collected en route.

In many towns and cities there are special health centres and dance/exercise classes for women. They're not always cheap, but they do ensure a regular routine (if you don't skip the classes!)

In addition to the specifically fitness-oriented exercises which we can do alone or with a group, there is one set of exercises—known as the Kegel exercises—which nearly all of us need to do regularly.

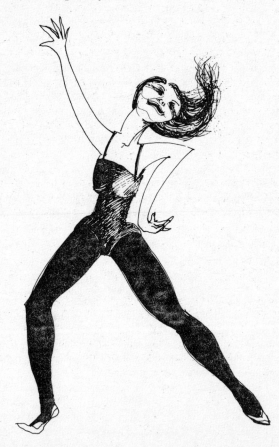

Maybe you like exercising to music.

Kegel exercises

These were designed in 1952 by a man called Arnold Kegel to help stress incontinence—that is, losing urine when you put strain on the set of muscles (called the PC muscle) around your pelvic area when you sneeze, cough, laugh or do exercises. This is an extremely common complaint, and a pretty embarrassing one for many of us. (One woman reported that her whole exercise class was put out of action by Star Jumps—and the resulting strain on so many out-of-tone PC muscles.) Like other muscles, this band of muscle, which is part of a string of muscles which stretch from your pubic bone to your tail bone, loses tone if not exercised regularly. As well as causing urine loss, a slack PC muscle can increase the likelihood of a prolapsed uterus (that is, the uterus literally falls well down into the vagina).

The hardest thing about the Kegel exercises is finding the muscle in the first place. The second most difficult thing is to remember to do them regularly, for to be of benefit they need to be done in small batches throughout the day. It is recommended that they be done in batches of five ten times daily: after two months you should notice a marked difference.

A physiotherapist who teaches the exercises explains: 'We tell our patients to do them each time they go near water, since running water often makes you want to urinate and reminds you of the need for them!'

Finding the muscle. Sit on the toilet with your legs well apart. Without moving your legs, try to stop the flow of urine. The PC muscle band is the one that controls the flow.

Exercise 1. Tighten the muscle, count to three, relax.
Exercise 2. Tighten and relax the PC muscle as quickly as you can.
Exercise 3. Pull up the whole pelvic floor ('like pushing your sleeves up', says the physiotherapist). Hold, then push down.

TEN

Cancer

It's tempting to try to shut our eyes to the whole subject of cancer—that's something that many of us do. The thought of contracting cancer is a scary one, certainly, but if we know how to detect the early signs we may have a fair chance of acting before the disease becomes life-threatening.

The three types of cancer which we particularly have to watch out for are cancer of the breast, cancer of the cervix (the neck of the uterus) and cancer of the uterus itself. Breast cancer is the single most common form to affect us; it is uncommon in the under 35 age group, but risks increase as we get older. It's important to realize that the disease is common enough to be taken seriously and that protective measures are simple, take up little of our time and cost nothing.

Those of us who are most at risk of breast cancer are women who:

- have a personal or family history of breast cancer
- have never had children
- have had a first child over the age of 30

There is a common myth that women who breastfeed are less at risk than those who don't. This theory has been discounted.

Breast cancer starts either in the ducts that take the milk to the nipple, or it begins further back, in the milk glands themselves. The cancer can then spread to the lymph nodes in the armpits or to those behind the breast bone. The sooner we detect the onset of the cancer, the less chance it will have to spread.

Ways to detect breast cancer

Self-examination is one of the best ways of detecting breast cancer. This should be done at the end of each period or, if you've stopped having periods, at regular monthly intervals. When doing a breast examination, you should be looking for changes which have occurred since the last time you examined yourself. After a while, you get used to the way your breasts look and feel, so these changes are easier to detect.

The chart below shows clearly how to feel for the changes. These can be in the overall size and shape of the nipple or breast; puckering of the nipple or the surrounding skin; a discharge from the nipple; changes in skin texture, or a swelling in your armpit or your upper arm. By looking in a mirror with your arms raised over your head, you'll be best able to see if any of these changes are happening.

After looking for the visible signs, the next thing to do is feel for any lumps or thickening. The lump may be soft or hard and may move slightly beneath your fingers. It may also be a soft, massy thickening over a whole area. You should also feel for any of these signs under your arms.

A low-dosage X-ray can sometimes detect breast cancer even before you can feel a lump. If you have any special concerns about breast cancer—for example, if your mother or sister has had breast cancer—your doctor can arrange for you to have a breast X-ray. It is recommended that all women over the age of 40 have a professional breast examination each year as well as doing regular self-examinations.

How to examine your breasts

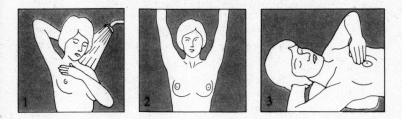

This simple three-step procedure could save your life by finding breast cancer early, at the stage when it is most curable.

1 *In the shower*. Examine your breasts during bath or shower; hands glide more easily over wet skin. Fingers flat, move gently but firmly over every part of each breast. Use right hand to examine left breast, left hand for right breast. Check for any lump, hard knot or thickening.
2 *Before a mirror*. Inspect your breasts with arms at your sides. Next raise your arms high over head. Look for: changes in size, shape or contour; bulging, swelling, puckering or dimpling; bleeding or discharge from the nipple; retraction or difference in height of the nipples.
3 *Lying down*. Lie on your back, putting a small pillow or towel under the right shoulder (this distributes the breast tissue evenly on the chest). Put your right hand behind your head.

Examine every area of the breast. Using the left hand and the flat of your fingers, press gently but firmly on the right breast, feeling for lumps. Work from the outer edge of the breast towards the nipple, a small area at a time, until you've worked around the whole breast with your fingers. (Think of your breast as a wheel with spokes.) Also feel the nipple area.

Do the same for the left breast, putting a towel under the left shoulder and with your left arm behind your head, feeling with the right hand. *The important thing is that you examine every area of the breast*.

When you should examine your breasts. The risk of breast cancer increases as you get older, but it's a good idea to begin monthly breast examination by the time you reach 25. Do it a few days after the menstrual period (before the period, many women have tender or 'lumpy' breasts). After menopause, choose a convenient day, such as the first of the month.

What you should do if you find a lump or thickening. If you find a lump or dimple or discharge, see your doctor as soon as possible. Don't be frightened. Most breast lumps or changes are *not* cancer, but only your doctor can decide if anything should be done.

Uterine cancer

Uterine cancer is a broad term for cancers that occur in the uterus (or the womb), and there are two parts of the uterus where a cancer begins.

The first is on the cervix or neck of the uterus. If you put your fingers in your vagina, you should be able to feel your cervix. Your uterus is a pear-shaped organ which is suspended by a piece of tissue across the top of your vagina. The second area in which a cancer may start is in the lining of the uterus, or endometrium, and is called endometrial cancer.

Cancer of the cervix

This occurs mainly in women over the age of 30. The symptoms to watch out for are vaginal bleeding after intercourse, pain during intercourse, unusual vaginal discharge and spotting between periods. If you've finished menopause, or have had your last period and then suddenly have another one months later, this too may be a potential sign of cancer which must be checked out by your doctor.

If cervical cancer is detected before it spreads beyond the cervix, the rate of cure is excellent. Regular smear tests should detect cell changes years before a true cancer develops and the smaller the cancer the better the rate of cure. Once the cancer has spread to neighbouring tissue or the lymph nodes, the outlook may not be as promising.

As a general rule every woman over 40 (and that means *every* woman) should have a cervical smear done once every three years. On reaching 65, further smears need not be taken from women who have had two consecutive negative smears. After that age there are few cases of cancer of the cervix detected in women who have been screened previously.

If you haven't had a cervical smear test, it simply involves a doctor's taking a small swab from the cervix and sending it to a laboratory for testing. It only takes a few seconds and doesn't hurt.

Endometrial cancer

Cancers of the body of the uterus occur mostly in women over the age of 45. Those of us most at risk are women who have had a late menopause (after 55) and women who have a combination of high blood pressure, diabetes and are overweight. The American Cancer Society also lists as risk factors a history of infertility, failure of ovulation and oestrogen therapy (but see also pp. 41–43).

The symptoms include any abnormal bleeding, bleeding between periods, a longer or heavier than normal flow of blood, and bleeding after your last period in menopause. (These can also be symptoms of fibroids—fibrous tumours which are very common and are non-malignant; they can be detected by pelvic examination.)

All women over the age of 40 should have a regular pelvic examination, during which your doctor will insert a finger into your vagina and with her or his other hand press down on your abdominal area to check your uterus, cervix, ovaries and Fallopian tubes. Cancer of the uterus can be detected by irregular bulk felt during the examination. Unhappily, cancer of the uterus cannot be detected simply by clinical examination. A specimen must always be taken from the lining of the womb for examination under the microscope.

If your doctor finds any symptoms or signs that suggest you may have endometrial cancer you will probably be advised to have what is known as a D and C (dilatation and curettage), which means that the inside of your uterus will be scraped and the scrapings examined for cancerous cells. A specimen from the lining of the womb can also be taken as an outpatient procedure using a special suction curette.

ELEVEN

How to Set Up Your Own Menopause Group

Some years ago I joined a consciousness-raising group. In that group we discussed all sorts of issues which we found difficult to deal with in our own lives. I found, much to my relief, that most of the issues which I thought were peculiar to me alone were shared by almost all the women in the group. It was helpful for me to hear the ways in which the other women had worked through particular issues and extremely reassuring to know that I wasn't the only one who harboured fears and self-doubts. Our group lasted for about two years, and although we no longer meet as a consciousness-raising group, we still get together regularly on a social basis. From that group I have made many close friends and have gained immense support through the rough patches of my life.

Our menopause sessions run on similar lines but look more specifically at the issues of menopause. During the 'factual' part of our sessions we talk about the physical experiences that our bodies may be going through, working on the theory that if we understand what's going on we're half way towards sorting out whether the things which are happening to us at menopause *are* based on physical changes or whether they are the result of more general, wider issues which we also need to look at.

Making changes can reap big rewards, and if we're thinking about changes it's very helpful to receive the support of others. The changes *don't* have to be big ones.

The main worth of the menopause sessions, though, is still the exchange of personal experiences. Over and over again women tell us how relieved they've been to find out what they were going through at menopause was shared by a large number of other women in the group. *Understanding what's going on is the first step to being able to do something positive about it.*

If you are interested in setting up a group of the kind I've talked about, it may be a good idea to see the menopause group as the starting point, for every menopause session I've ever been a part of has been so supportive and unthreatening that it's given us the confidence to look at some of the deeper subjects in more detail. The first time you run one, it may be a good idea to enlist the aid of a group of friends. And by trying out a session with a small group of no more than 12 people first, you'll be given the confidence to take on a larger session later.

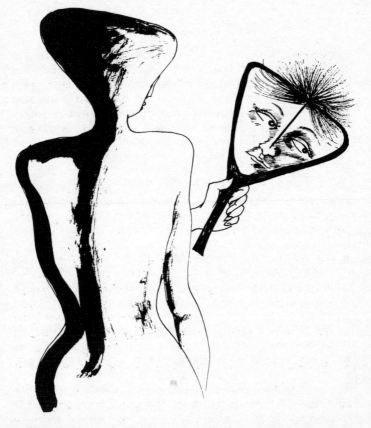

When we look at ourselves—at our fears and self-doubts—we often forget that other people feel those things too.

Arrange a time and date

The time you choose will largely depend upon the circumstances of the women who you hope will attend. Are women more likely to be free during the day, at night, or during the weekend? Bear in mind that the sessions will usually last for about three hours. That seems to be about right.

The date you choose should be somewhere from six to eight weeks in the future so that you have plenty of time to make the other arrangements without too much panic.

Arrange a venue

Community centres are often excellent venues as they are the focal point for many community activities. The ideal room is one which is quiet, private and large enough to hold 12 people comfortably. If possible, it should have tea-making facilities. Other suitable venues are private homes (as long as they have a room which is completely private), school rooms, public halls and some club rooms.

Advertise your session

Advertising may not be necessary if you are able to get together a group of women by word of mouth. If not, the sources of advertising below are all free:

- Make a poster or notice. This can be put in your local community centre, your local library and Citizens' Advice Bureau. You may be able to persuade local health centres, public health clinics, family planning clinics, doctors or chemists to display your notice, or you may be able to have it read out as a notice at any clubs you attend already.
- Write a small article for your local newspaper.

The personal column of newspapers is another outlet for advertising of groups. You will, however, have to pay for column space. In all advertising, remember to include the following details:

Time, date and length of session

Venue
Programme
Cost (if any)
Telephone number of pre-enrolment contact

Book women into your session

We have found that pre-enrolment of women into a session is essential so as to keep numbers at a manageable level. Don't be tempted to squeeze in more than 10 or 12 women.

If yours is the telephone number used for pre-enrolment, you need to be prepared to receive many calls, some of which will require a sympathetic ear. We find that it is wise to ensure that virtually everyone who comes to the sessions is actually going through menopause, for this makes the women feel free to discuss their problems.

You may wonder why we suggest restricting your sessions to women only. If this is the first chance that women have had to discuss menopause openly, women-only sessions are of much more benefit than mixed sessions. Most of us tend to be inhibited when talking about intimate experiences in the presence of men. Moreover, men are used to dominating conversation and discussion, and in our experience they tend to do this even in a session on menopause!

Find a professional

If you live in a city or large town, you may be able to get someone from a woman's health centre or family planning clinic to attend your session and to give out some of the factual information about menopause. But this is not essential. We have found that by far the greatest benefit of the sessions lies in our getting together to discuss the ways we are feeling. If you do get an outside speaker, make sure she is sympathetic to women going through menopause and is willing to answer questions.

Decide on cost

You may find it necessary to charge a small amount to cover speakers' travel expenses, tea and coffee (if needed) and the possible costs for hiring a room. Work out the appropriate sum and make sure that all the women attending know how much to pay in advance.

The day before the session

Recheck arrangements for getting into your venue, and make sure there are enough comfortable seats. Buy name labels, coffee, tea and biscuits, if you like. And make sure you have some money for change!

On the day of the session

Arrive early. Set up chairs in a circle (the best format for informal meetings); set up tea things and have a cup of tea ready for the women as they arrive. This tends to break the ice immediately.

When the women arrive, have them write their names on the labels you have provided and ask them to stick them somewhere visible on their clothing. (It's too difficult having to remember a room full of new faces *and* take in the talk.)

Have a tea break halfway through the session. This break is probably the most important and valuable part of the whole session, for it allows women to discuss their situation with those with whom they feel the most empathy. Allow the tea break to go on for as long as you feel is useful.

The session itself

Before you start the session, it's necessary to establish and state certain ground rules which will ensure that it runs smoothly and openly. The rules listed below have been developed with women who have attended our sessions. None of us can stress enough how important it is that they be adhered to.

- Women in the session must not judge or criticize others. They may be surprised or even shocked by what other women have to say, but this is not the place to express those feelings.

- What goes on is confidential. *Other people must not be discussed with anyone else outside the group.* This rule makes for a secure and non-threatening environment in which women will trust others and share their feelings.
- Interrupting others is not acceptable, and one or a few people must not be allowed to dominate. In a group where everyone is on an equal footing there is a much greater likelihood of open discussion taking place.

You will need to talk with the group about these ground rules before you begin talking about anything else. Once this has been done, you can move on to making introductions.

The woman (or women) who initiated the group may like to start the ball rolling by saying who they are and why they were prompted to set up the session in the first place. Then each woman in the group can introduce herself in turn and say what made her decide to come to the session. Introduce the guest speaker if there is one.

The main part

If you have a guest, ask her to begin by explaining very briefly the simple anatomical and hormonal aspects of the reproductive system. If you don't have a guest, one woman in the group could do this. All the information needed is in this book. You could even ask someone to read it out if no one feels confident enough to talk about it.

After this, you will probably find that the session takes off by itself if you go around the group talking about such issues as:

- How has menopause affected you physically—in other words, which physical symptoms have you had?
- Has menopause affected your feelings about your appearance? How?
- Has it affected your relationships with family and friends? In what ways?
- How has menopause affected your sexuality or relationships with sexual partners?
- What are some of the things you've discovered which have helped you cope with or overcome symptoms?

It may be an idea to have one of the women in the group primed to raise delicate issues, such as sexual needs or vaginal discharges, if it doesn't look as if anyone else is going to.

After the session

Women may want to exchange phone numbers and/or names of helpful books. You may also want to arrange to conttinue meeting as a health group or on a social basis.

One last word

As you have read, there is a lot you can do to help yourself improve your health and, hopefully, relieve some of your symptoms of menopause. There is also much to be gained from not 'going it alone'; the support and friendship of other women with similar experiences is invaluable.[29] All it takes is the initiative of one woman in the community to start the ball rolling.

Declaration of human rights[30]

You have the right:

- To express your own opinions, ideas and feelings.
- To disagree.
- To express the full range of emotion and feelings, including anger. (Without making excuses or apologizing.)
- To make your own decisions and to take responsibility for their consequences.
- To change your mind.
- To make mistakes and be responsible for them.
- To say 'I don't understand' or 'I don't know.'
- To say no without feeling guilty.
- To be independent of others, and to be dependent on others.
- To independent friendships.
- To have time entirely to yourself without being made to feel selfish.
- To ask and refuse help.
- To praise yourself.
- To .... YOU fill in.

References

Chapter 1
1   Richardson, R. G., *The Menopause: A Neglected Crisis*, Abbot Laboratories, Queensborough, Kent, NZ, 1973, p. 4.
2   Weideger, P., *Female Cycles*, The Women's Press Ltd, London, 1975, p. 205.

Chapter 2
3   Clay, V. S., *Women, Menopause and Middle Age*, Know Inc., Pittsburgh, Pennsylvania, 1977, p. 3.
4   Richardson, R. G., *ibid.*, p. 8.
5   *Ibid.*, p. 8.

Chapter 3
6   U.S. National Health Survey, in Dominian, J., 'The role of psychiatry in the menopause', *Clinics in Obstetrics and Gynaecology* 4 (1), 1977, pp. 241–57.
7   Clay, V. S., *ibid.*, pp. 22, 23, 46.
8   *Ibid.*, pp. 105–06.
9   Bolles, R., *What Colour is Your Parachute?* Ten Speed Press, Box 7123, Berkeley, California.
10 Abarbanl, K. and Siegel, C., *A Woman's Work Book*, Praeger, New York, 1975.
11 Boston Women's Health Book Collective, *Our Bodies Ourselves* (2nd Edition), Simon and Schuster, New York, 1976.
12 Dr Fothergill on 'The Management Proper at the Cessation of the Menses', in *Essays on Puerperal Fever and Other Diseases Peculiar to Women* (ed. Fleet and Churchill), 1849.
13 Galbraith, A. M., *The Four Epochs of Woman's Life*, W. B. Saunders and Co., 1904.
14 Tait, L., *Diseases of Women and Abdominal Surgery*, Vol. 1, Leicester, Richardson and Co., London, 1889, p. 152.
15 *Ibid.*, p. 153.

16   Editor's footnote to the article of Dr Fothergill, *ibid*.

17   Kelly, H. A., *Medical Gynaecology*, D. Appleton and Co., New York and London, 1908, pp. 151–53.

18   Fosberry, W. H. S., 'Severe climacteric flushings successfully treated'. Letter to the *British Medical Journal*, 24 April 1897, p. 1039.

19   Brown Sequard, C. E., 'On a new therapeutic method consisting in the use of organic liquids extracted from glands and other organs', *British Medical Journal*, 1, 1145–1147; 1212–1214, 1893.

20   Hutton, J. D., 'The Rational Use of Oestrogen in Menopause', *New Ethicals*, May 1981; 'Oestrogen Therapy after the Menopause: An Update on the Benefits vs. Risks', *New Ethicals*, March 1982.

Chapter 5
21   McWhirter, N. (ed.), *Guinness Book of World Records*, Sterling Publishing Co. Ltd., New York, 1981 and 1982, p. 29.

22   Seaman, B. and Seaman, G., *Women and the Crisis in Sex Hormones*, Bantam Books, 1977.

Chapter 6
23   Weideger, P., *Female Cycles*, The Women's Press Ltd., London, 1975, p. 205.

24   Kerr, C., *Sex for Women (Who Want to Have Fun and Loving Relationships with Equals)*, Grove Press, New York, 1978.

Chapter 7
25   Seaman, B. and Seaman, G., *ibid*.

Chapter 8
26   Spielberger, C., *Understanding Stress and Anxiety*, Harper and Row, New York, 1979.

27   Holmes, T. and Rahe, R., 'Holmes–Rahe Social Readjustment Rating Scale', *Journal of Psychosomatic Research*, 2, 1967.

Chapter 11
28   Butler, P., *Self Assertion for Women*, Harper and Row, 1976.

29 Smith, M. J., *When I Say No, I Feel Guilty*, Bantam Books, New York, 1975.
30 *Ibid.*

Index

Abortion 46, 50–51
Ageing 5–6, 29–30
Anaemia 74
Assertiveness training 89

Bloatedness 26
Breast cancer 96–98

Calcium 70–72, 74, 76–77
Carbohydrates 72
Cervical cancer 99
Climacteric 11

Depression 27, 29, 35, 43,
   78–79
Diet plan 79–80
Doctors 1–2, 19–20

Employment 31–33
Endometrial cancer
   99–100

Family Planning
   Association 6
Fats 72
Fertility 31
Flooding 25
Folate or Folic acid 73,
   75–76

Headaches 25
Hormones 14–18, 27, 39

Hormone treatments
   41–43
Hot flushes 11, 22–24,
   69, 77–78, 79
Hysterectomy 9, 44–45,
   49

Iron 74

Jogging 91–93

Kegel exercises 95

Libido 26

Masturbation 55–56, 65
Memory loss 26
Menopause group 6–7,
   36, 68, 101–107
Menstruation 3, 13,
   16–17, 30–31
Moods 11, 21, 27–28

Oestrogen 14–17, 25,
   41–43, 70
Osteoporosis 22, 25, 42,
   71
Ovaries 14–16

Parents 35
Progesterone 14–16, 42

Protein 71, 74
Puberty 17

Relationships 34–35
Relaxation 90

Smoking 13

Tubal ligation 49–50

Uterine cancer 99

Vaginal dryness 21, 24
Vasectomies 50
Vitamins 69, 73–75,
    78–79, 81

Weight gain 69, 77

Women and Depression
Deidre Sanders

A positive and practical guide for women and their families who want to understand depression, its causes, symptoms, the treatments prescribed and self-help remedies.   **£2.95**

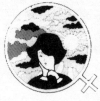

Women and Tranquillisers
Celia Haddon

A readable and intelligent guide to the different types of tranquillisers, their prescription, problems and side-effects. It is essential for anyone taking them or contemplating them.   **£2.95**

Eating Well for a Healthy Pregnancy
Dr Barbara Pickard

Ideal for all parents-to-be, it is a practical guide to eating before, during and after pregnancy to ensure a healthy baby. **£2.95**